T0260851

Examination of Peripheral Nerve Injuries

An Anatomical Approach

2nd Edition

Stephen Russell, MD
Assistant Professor
Department of Neurosurgery
Langone Medical Center
New York University
New York, NY

155 illustrations

Thieme
New York • Stuttgart • Delhi • Rio de Janeiro

Executive Editor: Timothy Hiscock
Managing Editor: Elizabeth Palumbo
Editorial Assistant: Mohammad Ibrar
Production Editor: Mason Brown
International Production Director: Andreas Schabert
Senior Vice President, Editorial and E-Product
Development: Cornelia Schulze
Senior Vice President and Chief Operating Officer:
Sarah Vanderbilt
President: Brian D. Scanlan

Library of Congress Cataloging-in-Publication Data

Russell, Stephen M., author.
  Examination of peripheral nerve injuries : an anatomical
approach / Stephen Russell. – Second edition.
    p. ; cm.
  Includes bibliographical references and index.
  Summary: "This book teaches the reader how to properly
examine a patient with a suspected focal neuropathy. This
instruction includes the pertinent anatomy of each peripheral
nerve, clear photographs illustrating the muscular examination,
and also discussion on how to approach localization and
diagnosis. Because a strong foundation in anatomical relationships is paramount for examining patients with nerve injury,
this is stressed in the text and by using numerous illustrations.
Readers can and will read the entire book and work to memorize
the more common problems and exams they will perform. They
will then consult it either before or after examining patients
with less common problems"–Provided by publisher.
  ISBN 978-1-62623-038-5 (softcover : alk. paper) – ISBN 978-
1-62623-039-2 (eISBN)
  I. Title.
  [DNLM: 1. Peripheral Nerve Injuries–diagnosis.
2. Peripheral Nerves–anatomy & histology. 3. Neurologic
Examination–methods. WL 530]
  RD595
  617.4'83–dc23
                                                    2014032048

© 2015 Thieme Medical Publishers, Inc.

Thieme Publishers New York
333 Seventh Avenue, New York, NY 10001 USA
+1 800 782 3488, customerservice@thieme.com

Thieme Publishers Stuttgart
Rüdigerstrasse 14, 70469 Stuttgart, Germany
+49 [0]711 8931 421, customerservice@thieme.de

Thieme Publishers Delhi
A-12, Second Floor, Sector-2, Noida-201301
Uttar Pradesh, India
+91 120 45 566 00, customerservice@thieme.in

Thieme Publishers Rio, Thieme Publicações Ltda.
Argentina Building 16th floor, Ala A,
228 Praia do Botafogo
Rio de Janeiro 22250-040 Brazil
+55 21 3736-3631

Cover design: Thieme Publishing Group
Typesetting by Thomson Digital, India

Printed in India by Replika Press Pvt. Ltd.   5 4 3 2 1

978-1-62623-038-5

Also available as an e-book:
978-1-62623-039-2

Important note: Medicine is an ever-changing science under-
going continual development. Research and clinical experience
are continually expanding our knowledge, in particular our
knowledge of proper treatment and drug therapy. Insofar as
this book mentions any dosage or application, readers may rest
assured that the authors, editors, and publishers have made
every effort to ensure that such references are in accordance
with **the state of knowledge at the time of production of the
book.**

Nevertheless, this does not involve, imply, or express any
guarantee or responsibility on the part of the publishers in
respect to any dosage instructions and forms of applications
stated in the book.

Every user is requested to examine carefully the manufacturers' leaflets accompanying each drug and to check, if neces-
sary in consultation with a physician or specialist, whether the
dosage schedules mentioned therein or the contraindications
stated by the manufacturers differ from the statements made in
the present book. Such examination is particularly important
with drugs that are either rarely used or have been newly
released on the market. Every dosage schedule or every form
of application used is entirely at the user's own risk and responsibility. The authors and publishers request every user to report
to the publishers any discrepancies or inaccuracies noticed. If
errors in this work are found after publication, errata will be
posted at www.thieme.com on the product description page.

Some of the product names, patents, and registered designs
referred to in this book are in fact registered trademarks or
proprietary names even though specific reference to this fact is
not always made in the text. Therefore, the appearance of a
name without designation as proprietary is not to be construed
as a representation by the publisher that it is in

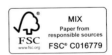

I dedicate this work to K.E.T.

Contents

Preface

The first edition has enjoyed a sustained popularity simply because it filled a niche in the medical literature that had theretofore been lacking—a concise description of both peripheral nerve anatomy and its physical examination. It was a resource for the seasoned practitioner, as well as a study guide for students and residents in a wide range of medical fields.

The strength of that monograph has been its focus. Therefore, we maintained that concentration when creating the second edition. The major improvements are in the schematics, which have been updated in collaboration with an illustrator. These new figures are not only aesthetically interesting, they are clearer and easier to understand. The text has also been systematically edited for clarity and flow.

Peripheral nerve anatomy and its physical examination provide one of the most beautiful and gratifying examples of form and its function in the human body. I hope you enjoy learning it!

1 Median Nerve

1.1 Anatomical Course

1.1.1 The Upper Arm

The median nerve (C6–T1) is derived from the lateral and medial cords of the brachial plexus, with the lateral cord providing mostly sensory axons from C6 and C7, and the medial cord mostly motor axons from C8 and T1. The brachial plexus cords receive their names (medial, lateral, and posterior) based on their relationship to the axillary artery underneath the pectoralis minor muscle. In agreement with this nomenclature, when viewing the upper arm from its medial (inside) surface toward the axilla, the medial cord is medial to the axillary artery and the lateral cord is lateral to the axillary artery. The terminal divisions of the medial and lateral cords merge to create the median nerve, forming a Y-shaped confluence over the superficial surface of the brachial artery.

The median nerve remains slightly lateral and superficial to the brachial artery as it travels down the arm. It runs anterior and parallel to the intermuscular septum, which separates the triceps from the flexors of the upper arm (i.e., biceps brachii, brachialis) (▶ Fig. 1.1). About halfway down the upper arm, the median nerve crosses over the top of the brachial artery, eventually resting just medial to it by the time it passes under the bicipital aponeurosis (lacertus fibrosis) in the proximal forearm. The median nerve innervates no muscles in the upper arm.

♦ **A few anatomical variations of the median nerve can occur in the upper arm. First, the medial and lateral cord components that form the median nerve may not fuse in the axilla, but instead join at a different point along the upper arm, sometimes as low as the elbow. Second, the medial and lateral cord components may loop under the axillary/ brachial artery prior to forming the median nerve. Finally, in some persons, the lateral cord contribution to the median nerve is very small, with the majority of the median nerve's C6 and C7 fibers running instead within the musculocutaneous nerve, only to be returned to the median nerve via a communication about halfway down the upper arm. This temporary misrouting of innervation is not an uncommon phenomenon; it is almost as if the fibers took a wrong turn during development, asked for some directions, and corrected themselves.**

1.1.2 The Antecubital Fossa/Elbow

The anatomy of the median nerve becomes more complex in the elbow region. It enters the antecubital fossa medial to the biceps brachii, passing over the brachialis muscle, which separates the nerve from the distal humerus. In

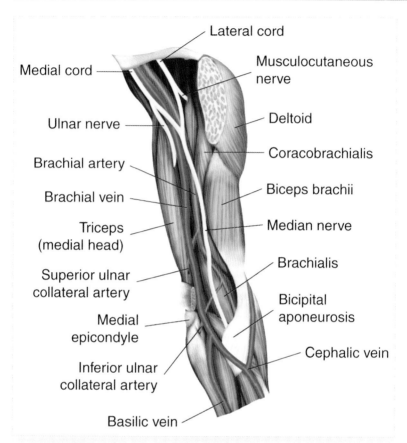

Fig. 1.1 Median nerve in upper arm. The median nerve remains slightly lateral and superficial to the brachial artery as it passes down the arm. About halfway down the arm, the median nerve crosses over the top of the brachial artery and then rests just medial to it by the time it passes under the bicipital aponeurosis.

the antecubital fossa, the median nerve passes under three successive arches or tunnels, eventually bringing it deep within the forearm, only for it to reemerge in the distal forearm prior to reaching the hand (▶ Fig. 1.2). The first arch it passes under is the bicipital aponeurosis (lacertus fibrosis), which is a thick layer of fascia attaching the biceps brachii to the proximal forearm flexor-pronator mass. Under this aponeurosis, the biceps tendon and brachial artery are both lateral to the median nerve, whereas the humeral head of the pronator teres muscle is medial (▶ Fig. 1.3). Of note, one may directly palpate the

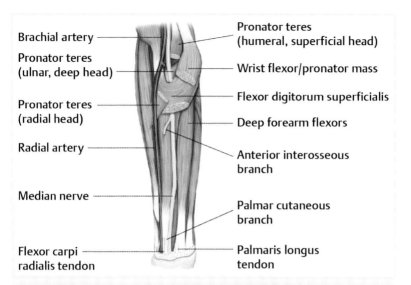

Brachial artery

Pronator teres (ulnar, deep head)

Pronator teres (radial head)

Radial artery

Median nerve

Flexor carpi radialis tendon

Pronator teres (humeral, superficial head)

Wrist flexor/pronator mass

Flexor digitorum superficialis

Deep forearm flexors

Anterior interosseous branch

Palmar cutaneous branch

Palmaris longus tendon

Fig. 1.2 Median nerve in the forearm. In the antecubital fossa, the median nerve passes under three successive arches or tunnels (bicipital aponeurosis [not shown], pronator teres [partially removed to expose the median nerve underneath], and flexor digitorum superficialis [under which the median nerve passes]), bringing it deep into the forearm, only for it to reemerge in the distal forearm prior to reaching the hand.

median nerve prior to its diving below this aponeurosis by palpating two fingerbreadths proximal, and two lateral, to the medial epicondyle.

A short distance past the proximal edge of the bicipital aponeurosis, the median nerve dives below a second structure—the humeral head of the pronator teres. The pronator teres is a Y-shaped muscle, with the bottom stem of the Y inserting into the radius, distal and lateral within the antecubital fossa. When viewing the antecubital fossa from anterior with the forearm supinated and extended, the Y of the pronator teres is turned on its side, so that the upper limbs of the Y are proximal, medial, and stacked on top of each other. These proximal two heads include a larger superficial head that attaches to the humerus (humeral head), and a deeper, smaller head that attaches to the ulna (ulnar head). The median nerve passes right in the crotch of this Y, with the ulnar head deep, and the humeral head superficial.

Next, just beyond the pronator teres, the median nerve almost immediately passes under a third structure: the two heads of the flexor digitorum superficialis (sublimis). This muscle's humeroulnar head is medial, whereas its radial head is lateral. The flexor digitorum superficialis, in essence, forms a second Y, through which the median nerve once again passes. In contrast to the pronator

3

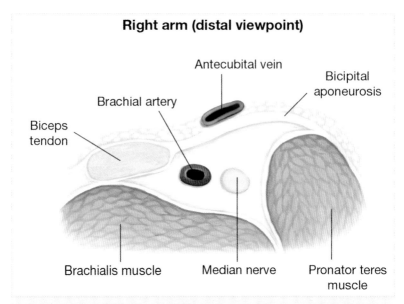

Right arm (distal viewpoint)

Antecubital vein

Bicipital aponeurosis

Brachial artery

Biceps tendon

Brachialis muscle   Median nerve   Pronator teres muscle

Fig. 1.3 Cross section of the median nerve in the antecubital fossa. The bicipital aponeurosis is superficial, the brachialis is deep, the biceps tendon and brachial artery are both lateral, and the humeral head of the pronator teres muscle is medial.

teres, however, when viewed anteriorly with the forearm supinated, the flexor digitorum superficialis's Y is not turned on its side. A fibrous ridge between its two heads is termed the sublimis ridge, and under this ridge, the median nerve passes. (I would suggest reviewing ▶ Fig. 1.2 and ▶ Fig. 1.20 and then rereading the preceding two paragraphs.)

◆ Variations in this area are usually musculotendinous. Either the prona- tor teres or the flexor digitorum superficialis may have only one head, not two, and their proximal origins may vary. These muscular varia- tions potentially create anatomical situations that may predispose the median nerve to entrapment within the antecubital fossa.

1.1.3 The Forearm

The median nerve travels down the center of the forearm deep to the flexor digitorum superficialis, but superficial to the underlying flexor digitorum profundus. More precisely, the median nerve lies toward the lateral margin of the flexor digitorum profundus, near the flexor pollicis longus, a muscle that lies just lateral to the flexor digitorum profundus. About one third to halfway down the forearm, an important branch of the median nerve, the *anterior interosseous nerve,* exits from its dorsolateral aspect. Once formed, the anterior interosseous nerve passes deeper within the forearm to run between the radius and ulna on the interosseous membrane, between and below the muscle bellies of the flexor digitorum profundus and flexor pollicis longus. This branch terminates in the distal forearm deep to the pronator quadratus. Near its origin, the anterior interosseous nerve passes under one or more fibrous ridges that originate off the pronator teres or flexor digitorum superficialis.

As the median nerve continues down the forearm it becomes superficial about 5 cm proximal to the wrist crease, just medial to the flexor carpi radialis tendon. When the wrist is flexed against resistance, the flexor carpi radialis tendon bowstrings proximal to the wrist. The median nerve is located just medial to this bowstrung tendon. The palmaris longus tendon, when present, lies just medial to the median nerve at the proximal wrist. Before entering the hand, the median nerve gives a pure sensory branch, the *palmar cutaneous branch,* which runs superficial to the carpal tunnel and ramifies over the proximal, radial half of the palm, particularly over the thenar eminence. Occasionally, this sensory branch passes through its own tunnel within the transverse carpal ligament.

The brachial artery also passes under the bicipital aponeurosis, where it bifurcates into the radial and ulnar arteries. The radial artery passes distally, near the superficial sensory radial nerve. The ulnar artery, alternatively, passes deep to the flexor-pronator muscle mass, where it loops under the median nerve. In the distal forearm, the ulnar artery joins the ulnar nerve, and together they travel toward the wrist. Prior to passing below the median nerve in the antecubital fossa, the ulnar artery gives the interosseous communis artery, which shortly thereafter divides into the anterior and posterior interosseous arteries. The anterior interosseous artery passes distally with the anterior interosseous nerve, deep between the flexor pollicis longus and flexor digitorum profundus.

1.1.4 The Wrist/Hand

The median nerve passes through the center of the wrist within the carpal tunnel. A common analogy is to think of the carpal tunnel as an upside-down table. The tabletop is composed of carpal bones, with the legs of the table being the hook of the hamate and pisiform medially, and the tubercle of the trapezium and distal pole of the scaphoid laterally. Stretched over these legs, like a rug on an imaginary floor, is the thick transverse carpal ligament. From a volar viewpoint, the median nerve is the most superficial of nine structures running through the carpal tunnel. These other structures include the flexor pollicis longus tendon, four superficial flexor tendons, and four deep flexor tendons (▶ Fig. 1.4). The palmaris longus tendon does not enter the carpal tunnel, but instead attaches more superficially to the palmaris aponeurosis. The flexor carpi radialis also does not pass through the carpal tunnel, but enters its own

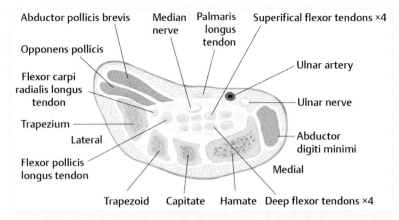

Fig. 1.4 Cross section of the median nerve in the carpal tunnel. The median nerve is the most superficial of nine structures running though the carpal tunnel. These other structures include the flexor pollicis longus tendon, four superficial flexor tendons, and four deep flexor tendons.

small tunnel, located lateral to the carpal tunnel, and attaches to the second metacarpal bone.

After passing through the carpal tunnel, the median nerve gives a branch off its radial side: the *thenar motor branch* (or recurrent thenar motor branch). Next, in the deep palm, the median nerve splits into two divisions: radial and ulnar. The radial division divides into the common digital nerve to the thumb and the proper digital nerve to the radial half of the index finger. The common digital nerve to the thumb subsequently divides into the two proper digital nerves to the thumb. The ulnar division of the median nerve divides into the common digital nerves of the second and third web spaces, which also subsequently divide into proper digital nerves. The ulnar and radial divisions of the median nerve run deep (i.e., dorsal) to the superficial palmar arterial arch, but superficial to the flexor tendons.

⬥ Numerous variations to the origin and path of the thenar motor branch can occur. For instance, it can prematurely originate within the carpal tunnel, it can pierce the transverse carpal ligament for a more direct route to the thenar muscles, and it can even emerge on the ulnar side of the median nerve, only to then cross deep or superficial to the median nerve to reach the thenar muscles. Other median nerve variations within the hand include (1) an early branching of the median nerve into radial and ulnar divisions proximal to the carpal tunnel (which often occurs with a "persistent median artery"), and (2) a connection between the thenar motor branch and the deep palmar branch of the ulnar nerve (discussion follows).

1.2 Motor Innervation and Testing

The median nerve does not innervate muscles in the upper arm. It does, how-ever, innervate numerous muscles in the forearm and hand that control fore-arm pronation, wrist flexion, flexion of the digits (especially the first three), and thumb opposition and abduction (▶ Fig. 1.5). To aid memorization, these muscles may be separated into four sequential groups: proximal forearm, ante-rior interosseous, thenar motor, and terminal.

1.2.1 The Proximal Forearm Group

Four muscles make up this group: pronator teres, flexor carpi radialis, flexor digitorum superficialis, and palmaris longus. The *pronator teres* (C6, C7) is the main pronator of the forearm and the first muscle innervated by the median nerve. Branches to the pronator teres exit the median nerve at the lowest aspect of the upper arm, prior to the median nerve passing between the two heads of the pronator teres. From a mechanical perspective, the elbow needs to be extended for the pronator teres to have mechanical advantage. Therefore, to test this muscle the elbow should be extended with the forearm fully pro-nated. The patient is then instructed to resist forced supination by the exam-iner (▶ Fig. 1.6).

The *flexor carpi radialis* (C6, C7) is one of the two major wrist flexors. The other is the *flexor carpi ulnaris,* which is innervated by the ulnar nerve. The flexor carpi radialis is the more important wrist flexor, however, with loss of function severely limiting wrist flexion except in an ulnar direction. Test the flexor carpi radialis by having the patient flex the wrist toward the anterior aspect of the forearm (i.e., not in the ulnar direction) (▶ Fig. 1.7). For patients with severe flexor carpi radialis weakness, have the patient flex the wrist with the forearm on a table, ulnar side down, which eliminates gravity. During wrist flexion the flexor carpi radialis tendon can be observed and palpated proximal to the wrist.

The *palmaris longus* (C7, C8) is attached to the palmar aponeurosis and cor-rugates the palmar skin. This muscle is not readily examined for muscular strength, and, in fact, is absent in about 15% of the population.

The *flexor digitorum superficialis* (known as the sublimis muscle, C8, T1) is also innervated by the median nerve. This muscle flexes the second through fifth digits (all except the thumb) at their proximal interphalangeal joints. To assess proximal interphalangeal joint flexion, each finger is tested separately. Placing your fingers between the patient's single finger to be tested and the remaining fingers isolates this movement (▶ Fig. 1.8). This maneuver places the finger to be tested in mild flexion at the metacarpal–phalangeal (knuckle) joint, and simultaneously stabilizes the remaining fingers in extension, a posi-tion that allows isolation of the flexor digitorum superficialis.

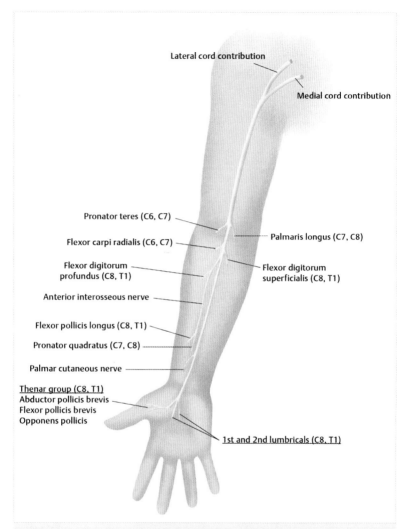

Fig. 1.5 Motor innervation of the median nerve. The median nerve does not innervate any muscles in the upper arm. It does, however, innervate numerous muscles in the forearm and hand that are involved in forearm pronation, wrist flexion, flexion of the digits (especially the first three), and thumb opposition and abduction.

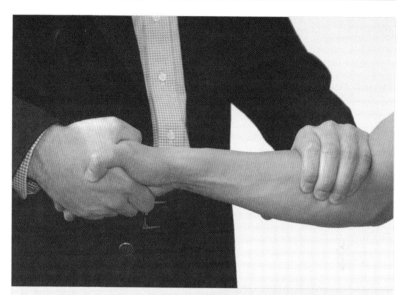

Fig. 1.6 Pronator teres (C6, C7) assessment: The patient's elbow is extended and the forearm is fully pronated. The patient is then instructed to resist supination of the forearm by the examiner.

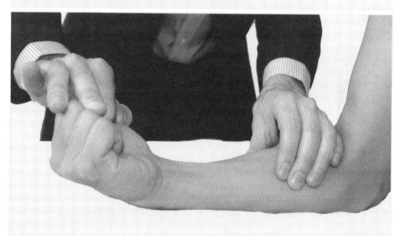

Fig. 1.7 Flexor carpi radialis (C6, C7) assessment: The patient flexes the wrist toward the anterior aspect of the forearm. For severe weakness, have the patient flex the wrist with the forearm on a table, ulnar side down, which eliminates gravity. Its tendon can be seen and palpated proximal to the wrist.

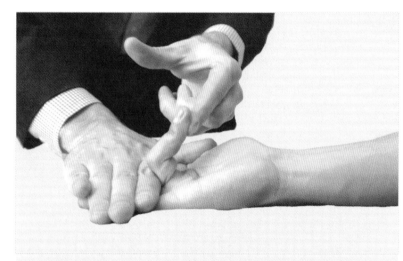

Fig. 1.8 Flexor digitorum superficialis (C8, T1) assessment: To test proximal inter-phalangeal joint flexion, the supinated forearm and hand are placed straight. Each finger is tested separately. Placing your fingers between the single finger to be tested and the remaining fingers that are immobilized isolates this movement. This maneuver places the finger to be tested in mild flexion at the metacarpal–phalangeal (knuckle) joint and stabilizes the remaining fingers in extension, a position that allows isolation of the flexor digitorum superficialis.

A topographical aid in identifying the muscles of the medial forearm flexor-pronator mass is to place a hand on the opposite forearm with its thenar eminence on the medial epicondyle, the ring finger along the medial border of the forearm, and the rest of the fingers naturally lying over the forearm pointing in a distal trajectory toward the other hand. In this position, the thumb is over the pronator teres, the index finger is over the flexor carpi radialis, the long finger is over the palmaris longus, and the ring finger is along the flexor carpi ulnaris, the latter being innervated by the ulnar nerve.

♦ When testing forearm pronation the patient should keep the fingers and hand relaxed to avoid supplemental pronation by the flexor carpi radialis and long finger flexors. When testing the finger flexors the wrist should be kept neutral and not allowed to extend because wrist extension causes passive finger flexion secondary to tenodesis. Tenodesis is movement at a distal joint (e.g., passive finger flexion) by lengthening the distance a tendon (e.g., a finger flexor tendon) has to pass by changing the position of a more proximal joint (e.g., wrist extension).

1.2.2 The Anterior Interosseous Group

The anterior interosseous nerve innervates three deeply situated anterior fore-arm muscles: the flexor digitorum profundus (to the second and third digits), the flexor pollicis longus, and the pronator quadratus. The *flexor digitorum profundus* (C8, T1), as a whole, is innervated by both the median and the ulnar nerves. The median nerve controls flexion of the distal interphalangeal joint of the second, and, partly, the third digits; the ulnar nerve controls this muscle's action upon the third (partly), fourth, and fifth digits. Distal interphalangeal joint flexion of the third (or long) digit has variable dominance by the median or ulnar nerves. Therefore, even with complete denervation of one of these nerves, some movement of the long finger is usually preserved because both the median and the ulnar portions of the flexor digitorum profundus act via a common tendon to this digit. To assess median innervation of the flexor digitorum profundus in isolation one should concentrate on the index finger. To do so, hold the metacarpal–phalangeal and proximal interphalangeal joints immobile and have the patient flex the distal phalanx against resistance (▶ Fig. 1.9).

The *flexor pollicis longus* (C8, T1) performs a function similar to the profundus but on the thumb; it flexes the distal phalanx of the thumb at the interphalangeal joint. Assess the flexor pollicis longus by immobilizing the thumb,

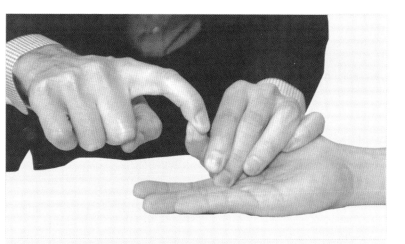

Fig. 1.9 Flexor digitorum profundus (C8, T1) assessment: To assess the median innervation of the flexor digitorum profundus one should concentrate on the index finger. To do so, hold both the metacarpal–phalangeal and proximal interphalangeal joints immobile and have the patient flex the distal phalanx against your resistance.

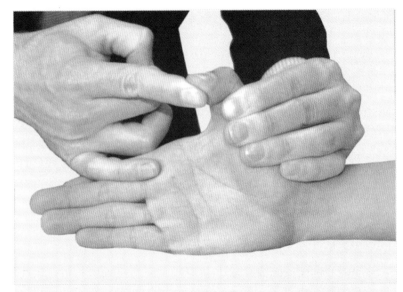

Fig. 1.10 Flexor pollicis longus (C8, T1) assessment: Immobilize the thumb, except the interphalangeal joint, and then ask the patient to flex the distal phalanx against resistance.

except the interphalangeal joint, and asking the patient to flex the distal phalanx against resistance (▶ Fig. 1.10). A quick way to assess both flexor digitorum profundus and flexor pollicis longus innervation from the anterior interosseous nerve is to ask the patient to make an okay sign by touching the tips of the thumb and index finger together. When these muscles are weak, the distal phalanges of the thumb and index finger cannot flex, and instead of the fingertips touching, the volar surfaces of each distal phalanx make contact (▶ Fig. 1.11).

The third muscle innervated by the anterior interosseous nerve is the *pronator quadratus* (C7, C8). This is a significantly weaker forearm pronator than the pronator teres. In fact, weakness of the pronator quadratus is often not readily apparent when the pronator teres is strong. However, fully flexing the forearm at the elbow removes the mechanical advantage of the pronator teres, and in this position weakness of the pronator quadratus should be detectable when compared with the normal arm (▶ Fig. 1.12).

◆ When testing the flexor digitorum profundus or the flexor pollicis longus, do not let the patient extend the distal interphalangeal joints beforehand because passive reflexion may mimic active joint flexion.

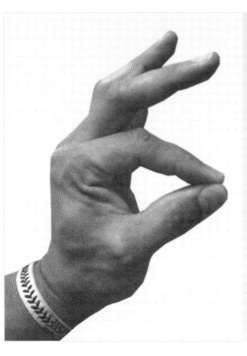

Fig. 1.11 "Okay" or "circle" sign with anterior interosseous nerve weakness. A quick way to assess the flexor digitorum profundus and flexor pollicis longus innervation from the anterior interosseous nerve is to ask the patient to make an okay sign by touching the tips of the thumb and index finger together. With weakness in these muscles, the distal phalanges cannot flex, and instead of the fingertips touching, the volar surfaces of each distal phalanx make contact.

1.2.3 The Thenar Group

The thenar group consists of three muscles innervated by the thenar motor branch of the median nerve. The first is the *abductor pollicis brevis* (C8, T1), which, as the name implies, abducts the thumb. There are two types of thumb abduction: palmar abduction away from the plane of the palm (mediated by the abductor pollicis brevis), and radial abduction away from the line of the forearm (mediated by the abductor pollicis longus). Therefore, even with a complete palsy of the abductor pollicis brevis, radial abduction of the thumb can still occur. To test the abductor pollicis brevis, resist movement of the thumb away from the plane of the palm (palmar abduction) while the hand is immobilized (▶ Fig. 1.13).

Next, the *flexor pollicis brevis* (C8, T1) has both a deep and a superficial head. It is innervated by both the median nerve (its superficial head) and the ulnar nerve (its deep head). This muscle flexes the thumb at the metacarpal–phalangeal joint. To test the flexor pollicis brevis, immobilize the thumb's interphalangeal joint and have the patient flex at the metacarpal–phalangeal joint (▶ Fig. 1.14). Make certain the distal interphalangeal joint does not flex,

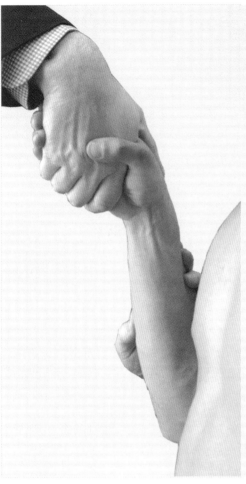

Fig. 1.12 Pronator quadratus (C7, C8) assessment: Have the patient resist supination with the elbow fully flexed and the forearm pronated. With full flexion at the elbow, pronation by the usually dominant pronator teres is minimized.

because, if this is allowed, substitution by the flexor pollicis longus may occur. Furthermore, use your other hand to immobilize the first metacarpal (i.e., immobilize the palm) to reduce substitution by the opponens pollicis. Because the flexor pollicis brevis is dually innervated, some thumb flexion can still occur following a complete median nerve injury. Nevertheless, when compared with the normal hand, weakness is usually apparent.

Assess the *opponens pollicis* (C8, T1) by having the patient forcibly maintain contact between the volar pads of the distal thumb and fifth digit while you try to pull the distal first metacarpal away from the fifth digit (► Fig. 1.15).

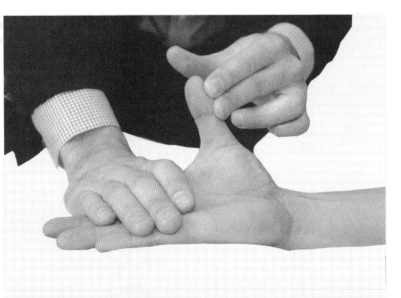

Fig. 1.13 Abductor pollicis brevis (C8, T1) assessment: Resist movement of the thumb away from the plane of the palm (palmar abduction), while stabilizing the metacarpals of the remaining fingers.

Although the median nerve independently controls thumb opposition, a combination of thumb adduction (adductor pollicis; ulnar nerve) and thumb flexion (flexor pollicis brevis; deep head, ulnar nerve) may mimic thumb opposition when a complete median nerve palsy is present.

◆ **Examining the motor function of the thumb is not straightforward. The key principle is to compare the results with the normal hand, keeping in mind that, even after complete loss of median nerve function, some movement of the thumb may occur secondary to either true muscle action via radial and ulnar innervation or substitutions by adjacent muscles.**

1.2.4 The Terminal Group

The terminal group simply consists of the *first and second lumbricals* (C8, T1), which are innervated by the terminal radial and ulnar divisions of the median nerve, respectively. To examine the first lumbrical, stabilize the index finger in a hyperextended position at the metacarpal–phalangeal joint and then provide

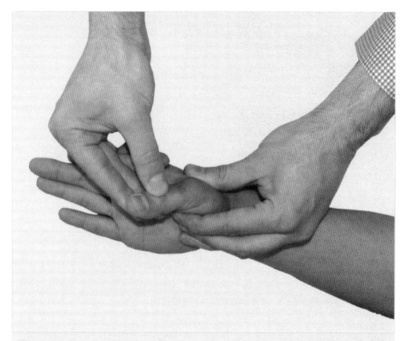

Fig. 1.14 Flexor pollicis brevis (C8, T1) assessment: The patient flexes the thumb at the metacarpal–phalangeal joint against resistance placed over both the proximal and the distal phalanges. Make certain that the distal interphalangeal joint does not flex because, in allowing this, substitution by the flexor pollicis longus occurs. Use your other hand to immobilize the first metacarpal to reduce substitution by the opponens pollicis. Because of its dual innervation, even with complete thenar motor branch palsies some thumb flexion still occurs.

resistance as the patient extends the finger at the proximal interphalangeal joint (▶ Fig. 1.16).

◆ The muscular origins and insertions of the lumbricals are quite variable. In fact, one or more lumbricals may be absent. This variability or absence of the lumbricals is functionally acceptable because flexion at the metacarpal–phalangeal joints and extension at the proximal interphalangeal joints when the metacarpal–phalangeal joints are hyperextended (both movements performed by the lumbricals) are also partly performed by the palmar and dorsal interossei muscles. Keep in mind that, whenever you test lumbrical strength, they are being assisted by the interossei.

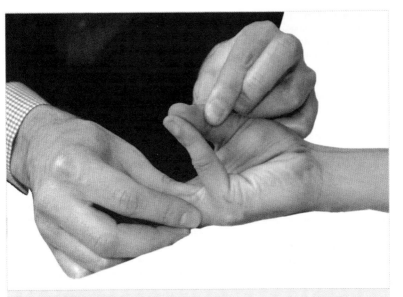

Fig. 1.15 Opponens pollicis (C8, T1) assessment: Have the patient forcibly maintain contact between the volar pads of the distal thumb and fifth digit, while you try to pull the distal first metacarpal away from the fifth digit. Although thumb opposition is only innervated by the median nerve, a combination of thumb adduction (adductor pollicis; ulnar nerve) and thumb flexion (flexor pollicis brevis, deep head, ulnar nerve) may mimic thumb opposition even when there is complete denervation of the opponens pollicis.

1.3 Sensory Innervation

The median nerve provides sensation to a vital region of the hand. Via three branches, the *palmar cutaneous nerve* and the *radial and ulnar divisions of the median nerve* (via digital branches) in the palm, the median nerve carries cutaneous sensory information from the radial two thirds of the palm and the volar surfaces of the first, second, third, and radial half of the fourth digits (▶ Fig. 1.17). Dorsal fingertip sensation is also carried by the median nerve, including the dorsum of the ulnar half of the distal phalanx of the thumb. The palmar cutaneous branch innervates the majority of the median nerve's palmar distribution, whereas sensation from the fingers is through branches of the median nerve's radial and ulnar divisions in the palm. Therefore, one should use the thenar eminence to assess the palmar cutaneous branch, and the distal portion of the second and third digits to assess the sensory fibers that pass through the carpal tunnel. In addition to sensory cutaneous

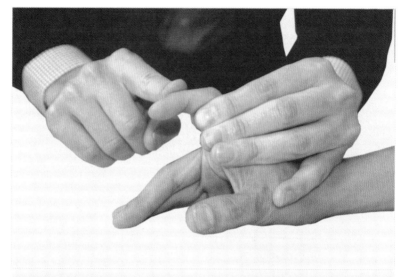

Fig. 1.16 Lumbrical of second digit (C8, T1) assessment: Stabilize the patient's index finger in a hyperextended position at the metacarpal–phalangeal joint and then provide resistance as the patient extends the finger at the proximal interphalangeal joint.

innervation, the median nerve also carries sensory fibers for joint proprioception and muscle tension, especially from the elbow and wrist. Although many refer to the anterior interosseous nerve as a "pure" motor nerve without cutaneous innervation, it does, in fact, carry sensory fibers from the wrist joints as well as from the muscles it innervates.

♦ The ulnar border of the median nerve's sensory innervation on the hand may vary depending on its relationship, or dominance over, the adjacent ulnar nerve. For example, either the ulnar or the median nerve may receive sensory innervation from the complete volar fourth digit. Furthermore, the percentage of the palm's median nerve–innervated region carried by the palmar cutaneous branch versus branches of the radial and ulnar divisions of the median nerve can also be variable.

1.3.1 Martin-Gruber and Riche-Cannieu Anastomoses

Cross talk, or anastomoses, between the ulnar nerve and either the median nerve or its anterior interosseous branch may occur in the forearm. Many variations are possible, and knowing a few of the more common ones is clinically useful.

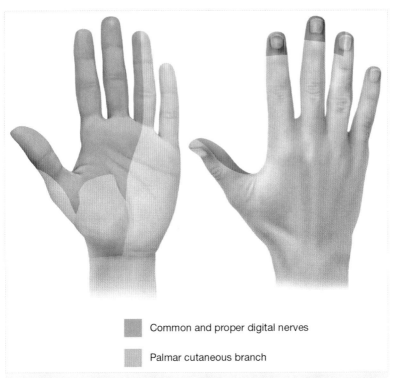

Common and proper digital nerves

Palmar cutaneous branch

Fig. 1.17 Sensory innervation of the median nerve. The median nerve carries cutaneous sensory information from the radial two thirds of the palm, and the volar surfaces of the first, second, third, and radial half of the fourth digit.

The *Martin-Gruber anastomosis* occurs in up to 15% of patients and involves the median innervated thenar muscles (opponens pollicis, abductor pollicis brevis, and flexor pollicis brevis). In this anomaly, instead of their usual pathway down the median nerve and out the thenar motor branch, nerve fibers destined for these three muscles instead run down the anterior interosseous branch, are subsequently transferred to the ulnar nerve in and around the flexor digitorum profundus muscle, and then enter the palm via the deep branch of the ulnar nerve. Within the palm, these fibers are eventually transferred back to the thenar motor branch, where they innervate their respective muscles. This distal communication between the deep ulnar branch and the thenar motor branch in the palm is termed the *Riche-Cannieu anastomosis*.

Therefore, when motor axons destined for the median nerve's thenar muscles cross over to the ulnar nerve via the Martin-Gruber anastomosis, low median nerve injuries in the wrist or forearm can paradoxically spare thenar motor function. The corollary is that damage to the ulnar nerve near the wrist in these patients can cause a more severe deficit of intrinsic hand function than expected.

◆ **Another version of the Martin-Gruber anastomosis involves the hand intrinsic muscles usually innervated by the deep branch of the ulnar nerve in the hand, including the lumbricals, first dorsal interosseous, adductor pollicis, and deep (ulnar) portion of the flexor pollicis brevis. For this variation, motor axons innervating these muscles accidentally pass down the median nerve and then pass back to the ulnar nerve halfway down the forearm via communications with the anterior interosseous branch of the median nerve, through or around the flexor digitorum profundus muscle. Yet another variation is when the median nerve's thenar motor branch aberrantly innervates the third lumbrical, or even all the lumbricals, via the Riche-Cannieu anastomosis.**

1.4 Clinical Findings and Syndromes

1.4.1 The Upper Arm

Complete Palsy

Damage to the median nerve in the arm is usually secondary to trauma: lacerations, gunshots, or blunt contusions. Because of the median nerve's close proximity to the brachial artery, concomitant injury to this vessel may occur. In the proximal upper arm both the ulnar and the radial nerves are in close proximity to the median nerve, and, therefore, all three of these nerves can be simultaneously injured *(triad neuropathy)*. Pressure palsies, like the *Saturday night palsy,* which can occur from hanging the arm over the back of a chair and passing out (e.g., when intoxicated), or the *honeymooner's palsy,* which occurs when your arm is under the neck of your partner sleeping next to you for a length of time, can injure the median nerve. Although it usually injures the radial nerve, the head of a crutch can also damage the median nerve in the axilla.

A complete injury to the median nerve is debilitating. Numbness occurs on the volar surfaces of the first three and a half digits and the radial two thirds of the palm. The forearm cannot pronate against gravity or resistance. The hand can only weakly flex at the wrist in an ulnar direction. The thumb cannot be opposed or abducted in a palmar direction. Lumbrical weakness in the index

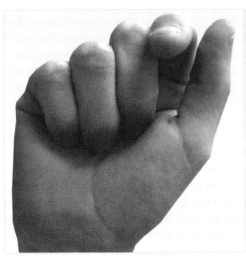

Fig. 1.18 Benedictine sign. When a patient with a complete median palsy is asked to make a fist, the first digit (i.e., the thumb) barely flexes, the second digit partially flexes (secondary to substitution from non–median innervated muscles), the third digit flexes but is weak, while the fourth and fifth digits flex normally, creating what is known as the Benedictine sign.

and long fingers is present. Additionally, when a patient with a complete median palsy is asked to make a fist, the first digit barely flexes, the second digit partially flexes (secondary to substitution from non–median innervated muscles), the third digit flexes but is weak, while the fourth and fifth digits flex normally, which is called a *Benedictine sign* (or *orator's hand*) (▶ Fig. 1.18). This sign of median nerve palsy is so named because of its similarity to the hand position during blessings, and is seen in many paintings of Jesus.

When examining a complete median nerve palsy, the following pitfalls must be considered. The brachioradialis (innervated by the radial nerve), with the help of gravity, may pronate the forearm from full supination. Next, you may observe thumb opposition by the indirect actions of the flexor pollicis brevis (its deep muscle head) and the adductor pollicis (both innervated by the ulnar nerve).

Supracondylar Spur/Ligament of Struthers

Rarely, people can have a supracondylar spur on the medial side of the humerus, about 5 cm proximal to the medial epicondyle. When this accessory condyle is present a ligament bridging it to the medial epicondyle frequently occurs. This ligament is called the *ligament of Struthers* after the anatomist who first described the supracondylar spur. When present, the median nerve usually passes underneath this ligament with either the brachial artery or its ulnar artery branch. This anatomically confined channel can cause median nerve entrapment in some patients (▶ Fig. 1.19).

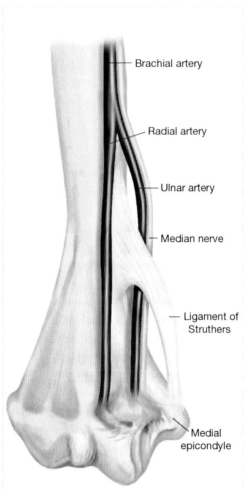

Fig. 1.19 Ligament of Struthers. Approximately 1% of people have a supracondylar spur on the medial side of the humerus about 5 cm proximal to the medial epicondyle. When this accessory condyle is present, in most cases there is a ligament bridging this supracondylar spur to the medial epicondyle.

Brachial artery

Radial artery

Ulnar artery

Median nerve

Ligament of Struthers

Medial epicondyle

Clinically, this entrapment has been reported to cause insidious onset of forearm and hand weakness, with variable sensory loss in a median distribution. A deep aching pain is often present in the proximal forearm, which occasionally worsens with repetitive pronation/supination, or during strength testing of the pronator teres or flexor carpi radialis. On examination, weakness, and even muscle wasting, may occur in any median nerve–innervated muscle. The branches to the pronator teres can sometimes arise proximal to where the median nerve passes under the ligament of Struthers. In this case the pronator teres would be spared. Although a rare diagnosis, all patients with more distal median nerve palsies (e.g., carpal tunnel syndrome) should have their wrist and finger flexors tested, including the muscles innervated by the anterior interosseous nerve, to exclude this more proximal entrapment. A Tinel sign in the distal, medial upper arm may be present. Of course, palpation or a radiograph confirming the presence of a supracondylar spur is also required to make this diagnosis.

Supracondylar Fractures

Supracondylar fractures usually occur in children and may cause median nerve damage. This is especially true for displaced fractures. Delayed median palsies can also occur secondary to progressive callus formation or misalignment. Traumatic supracondylar injuries often involve axons destined for the anterior interosseous nerve. This occurs for two reasons. First, the relatively fixed anterior interosseous nerve is placed on stretch when a fractured arm is displaced posteriorly. Second, the nerve fibers destined for the anterior interosseous nerve, along with the sensory fibers destined for the first two digits, are located posteriorly in the median nerve and are prone to injury from a supracondylar fracture. When a patient has isolated anterior interosseous motor loss secondary to partial median nerve damage in the supracondylar region (i.e., not direct damage to the anterior interosseous nerve), this injury is called a *pseudo–anterior interosseous neuropathy*. Often, patients with this type of neuropathy have some thumb and index finger numbness, which can help differentiate this injury from a true anterior interosseous nerve palsy.

1.4.2 The Forearm

Musculotendinous Median Neuropathies

The bicipital aponeurosis, which crosses from lateral to medial over the antecubital fossa and serves to attach the biceps brachii tendon indirectly to the ulna, may irritate the median nerve. The pathogenesis of this is uncertain, but a thickened aponeurosis, hypertrophied brachialis (which lies under the median nerve and theoretically can displace it against the bicipital aponeurosis), or an anomalous muscle insertion of the pronator teres (which alters the local anatomical arrangements) may each predispose to this type of compression. Patients with bicipital aponeurosis entrapment have a similar presentation and exam to those with ligament of Struthers compression. They frequently report elbow pain radiating both proximally and distally. Occasionally, resisted forearm flexion in the supinated position for 30 seconds may precipitate symptoms. Of note, this compression is very rare.

23

The median nerve may be compressed or pinched where it passes between the two heads of the pronator teres (▶ Fig. 1.20). This occurs most commonly in people who perform repetitive, forceful pronation of their forearm; it is called *pronator teres syndrome.* The only median-innervated muscle that is not affected by this syndrome is the pronator teres itself. This is because branches from the median nerve destined for this muscle originate proximal to where the median nerve passes underneath it. Pronator teres syndrome is characterized by an insidious onset of dull aching pain in the proximal forearm that is worsened by repetitive or forceful pronation. In fact, the most common finding is tenderness of the pronator teres to palpation. Median-innervated hand sensation is often normal, and motor function may be difficult to ascertain because of pain. Nonetheless, weakness is occasionally seen during flexion of the second and third digits. A Tinel sign can often be elicited at the antecubital fossa. In contradistinction to carpal tunnel syndrome, patients usually do not complain of nocturnal pain or numbness. The true incidence of this syndrome is unknown, and some authors suggest it should be separated into those with objective findings versus those without.

A fibrotic arch between the two heads of the flexor digitorum superficialis may also irritate the median nerve (▶ Fig. 1.20). This ridge has been called the *sublimis arch,* and it may compress the median nerve as it passes underneath. Clinical manifestation of this entrapment is quite similar to that of pronator teres syndrome, except that forceful flexion of the proximal interphalangeal joints of the second to fifth digits, which is mediated by contraction of the flexor digitorum superficialis muscle, may precipitate symptoms.

Of note, with surgical treatment of median nerve entrapment at the elbow, all three possible compression points—bicipital aponeurosis, pronator teres, and sublimis arch—are each inspected and decompressed.

The Anterior Interosseous Nerve

An isolated palsy affecting the anterior interosseous nerve may occur secondary to trauma, fractures, Parsonage-Turner syndrome, anomalous muscles and/ or tendons, or without a known cause. Patients usually complain of weakness or clumsiness in grasping objects with their first two digits (e.g., grasping the handle of a coffee cup). There are usually no complaints of pain, and because this nerve does not carry cutaneous sensation, no numbness occurs. There is weakness of the flexor digitorum profundus (to the second and third digits), flexor pollicis longus, and pronator quadratus. Patients have a positive okay sign (▶ Fig. 1.11). To confirm a pure, anterior interosseous nerve palsy, all other median nerve–innervated muscles, as well as sensation, must be normal. Partial anterior interosseous palsies are possible, as are partial median nerve palsies mimicking an anterior interosseous nerve deficit (e.g., pseudo–anterior interosseous neuropathy). Although anterior interosseous nerve palsy is a clin-

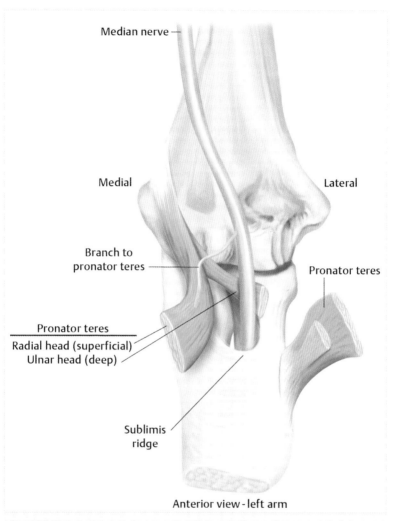

Median nerve

Medial

Lateral

Branch to
pronator teres

Pronator teres

Pronator teres
Radial head (superficial)
Ulnar head (deep)

Sublimis
ridge

Anterior view - left arm

Fig. 1.20 Pronator teres syndrome and sublimis arch. The median nerve may be compressed or pinched where it passes between the two heads of the pronator teres. A fibrotic arch may alternatively compress it when it passes under the two heads of the flexor digitorum superficialis.

ical diagnosis, magnetic resonance imaging (MRI) would show denervation of the three muscles innervated by this nerve.

⬥ **Patients with rheumatoid arthritis can have spontaneous and painless rupture of the flexor digitorum profundus and flexor pollicis longus tendons, mimicking an anterior interosseous palsy. To exclude this possibility, have the patient open and relax the hand. If the tendons are intact, pressing your thumb firmly across the ventral aspect of the forearm about 2 to 3 inches proximal to the wrist should cause passive finger flexion.**

1.4.3 Carpal Tunnel Syndrome

The symptoms of carpal tunnel syndrome are well described: aching pain and paresthesias in the radial half of the palm and first three digits that wakes the patient up at night and is relieved by "shaking it away." Of course, each patient's presentation is a variation of this central theme; perhaps it is only in the fingers, maybe the patient doesn't "shake it away," maybe it is only paresthesias or coldness, and so on. On examination, hypesthesia, hyperesthesia, and/or diminished vibratory sense may be present in the first three digits. Remember, the majority of median innervated palm sensation is via the palmar cutaneous branch, which does not pass through the carpal tunnel. Therefore, objective sensory testing on the thenar eminence should be, and usually is, normal; nevertheless, patients commonly report pain and "abnormal" sensation in this area. In severe cases, thenar muscle wasting can be seen, as well as weakness in thumb opposition, flexion, and palmar abduction. Rarely, the thenar motor branch is selectively compressed. Other tests include a Tinel sign at the wrist, the Phalen test, and the reverse Phalen test. A Phalen test is positive when flexing the affected wrist for about 1 minute precipitates symptoms. In a reverse Phalen test extending the wrist has the same effect.

Space-occupying lesions (e.g., ganglion cysts, anomalous lumbrical muscles, fractures, etc.) in the carpal tunnel may predispose one to this syndrome. Certain systemic diseases are also associated with entrapment here, including diabetes, chronic dialysis treatment, rheumatoid arthritis, acromegaly, obesity, and hypothyroidism, to name a few. A genetic predisposition to carpal tunnel syndrome (familial carpal tunnel syndrome) has also been reported; these patients are thought to have a small carpal tunnel and/or a thickened transverse carpal ligament.

A simple grading system separating carpal tunnel syndrome into mild, moderate, and severe is useful for treatment decision making and prognosis. *Mild* carpal tunnel syndrome includes complaints of numbness and tingling at night and occasionally during the day. The most common area involved is the long finger followed by the palm. A significant portion of the day the patient's hand feels almost normal. Pain is uncommon at this early stage. Two-point discrimination is usually okay, although vibration sense and light touch may actually be heightened in the affected fingers. No weakness or atrophy is present. In *moderate* carpal tunnel syndrome, the symptoms are more pervasive throughout the day. Sensory testing now reveals hypesthesia to light touch and vibration. Two-point discrimination may be abnormal. A Tinel sign is now present at the wrist, and a Phalen test may be positive. Muscle weakness is still not present. In *severe* carpal tunnel syndrome, the patient's symptoms are constant, weakness and atrophy may occur, and a Tinel sign at this point may even be absent secondary to extensive nerve damage. To reiterate, mild carpal tunnel syndrome is a diagnosis of medical history, with physical findings not usually present; moderate cases have sensory abnormalities and likely a Tinel sign; and severe cases have constant sensory symptoms and perhaps motor weakness.

2 Ulnar Nerve

2.1 Anatomical Course

2.1.1 The Arm

After the medial cord's contribution to the median nerve, it continues distally as the ulnar nerve. The ulnar nerve is predominantly made up of fibers from the C8 and T1 spinal nerves. However, C7 input may also be present (to be discussed).

The transformation of the medial and lateral cords into their terminal branches is M-shaped, lying over the anterior aspect of the axillary artery. The lateral leg of the letter M is the musculocutaneous nerve; the medial leg is the ulnar nerve. The center, V-shaped, convergence is the lateral and medial cords merging to become the median nerve (▶ Fig. 2.1).

Before the medial cord becomes the ulnar nerve, it yields two important sensory branches, the *medial brachial cutaneous* and *medial antebrachial cutaneous* nerves, which innervate the medial half of the upper arm and forearm, respectively (▶ Fig. 2.2). Therefore, sensory loss involving these two nerves would help localize an injury proximal to the ulnar nerve.

The medial brachial cutaneous nerve pierces the superficial fascia of the arm near the axilla and subsequently passes in the subcutaneous space innervating the medial surface of the upper arm. The distal portion of this nerve may reach an area posterior to the medial epicondyle; in this region it may be inadvertently transected during ulnar nerve decompressions.

The medial antebrachial cutaneous nerve branches into an anterior and posterior branch just proximal, and anterior to, the medial epicondyle. Near this bifurcation, components of these branches pierce the superficial fascia of the arm and enter the subcutaneous space. The anterior division runs along the anteromedial forearm, whereas the posterior branch runs along the posteromedial aspect of the forearm. The posterior branch *often* crosses the operative field for decompression of the ulnar nerve, where it may be injured during surgery. The anterior branch can be harmed when the median nerve is exposed in the antecubital fossa.

In the proximal upper arm, the ulnar nerve runs along the brachial artery's medial aspect, opposite the median nerve, which runs on the brachial artery's lateral side (▶ Fig. 2.3). Here, the ulnar nerve lies on the anterior border of the intermuscular septum, a thick fascial plane that separates the flexor and extensor compartments of the arm. At about the coracobrachialis muscle's insertion into the humerus, which occurs halfway down the upper arm, the ulnar nerve pierces this intermuscular septum. The superior ulnar collateral artery, a branch from the brachial artery, runs with the ulnar nerve through

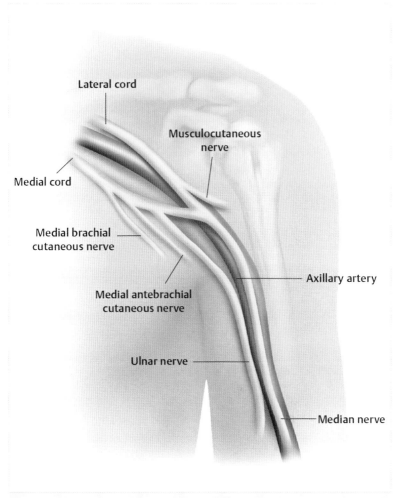

Fig. 2.1 Origin of the ulnar nerve in the axilla. The transformation of the medial and lateral cords into their terminal branches is M-shaped, lying over the anterior aspect of the axillary artery. The lateral leg of the letter M is the musculocutaneous nerve; the medial leg is the ulnar nerve. The center, V-shaped convergence is the lateral and medial cords merging to become the median nerve.

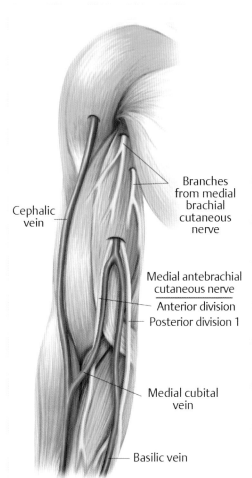

Fig. 2.2 Course of the medial brachial and antebrachial cutaneous nerves. Before the medial cord becomes the ulnar nerve, it yields two important sensory branches, the medial brachial cutaneous and the medial antebrachial cutaneous nerves, which innervate the medial half of the arm and forearm, respectively.

Cephalic vein

Branches from medial brachial cutaneous nerve

Medial antebrachial cutaneous nerve
Anterior division
Posterior division 1

Medial cubital vein

Basilic vein

Right arm, anterior view

this septum. Once piercing the intermuscular septum, the ulnar nerve becomes enveloped in the anteromedial aspect of the medial head of the triceps, inside of which it continues down the arm. In about 50% of the general population, an extension of the intermuscular septum forms an arch, or arcade, that attaches to the medial head of the triceps. This structure is a few centimeters in length and is located about two thirds of the way down the arm. It is called the *arcade of Struthers*. The ulnar nerve, which is deep and enveloped in the medial

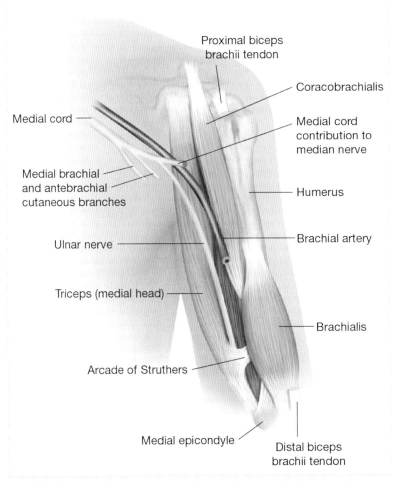

Fig. 2.3 The course of the ulnar nerve in the arm. In the proximal upper arm, the ulnar nerve lies on the anterior border of the intermuscular septum. Once piercing the intermuscular septum, the ulnar nerve becomes enveloped in the anteromedial aspect of the medial head of the triceps.

triceps head, would run under this arcade, when present. The arcade of Struthers should not be confused with the ligament of Struthers, which bridges an anomalous supracondylar ridge on the distal humeral shaft to the medial humeral epicondyle (see Chapter 1, Median Nerve). As the medial head of the triceps narrows into its distal tendon, the ulnar nerve emerges from its passage within this muscle and enters the posteromedial elbow region. The inferior ulnar artery, which also arises from the brachial artery, joins the ulnar nerve here. Branches of the inferior ulnar artery adhere to, and pass with, the ulnar nerve through the elbow region.

The mobility of the ulnar nerve changes as it passes down the medial arm. When anterior to the intermuscular septum in the upper half of the arm the ulnar nerve is mobile. However, it subsequently becomes immobilized in the lower half of the arm by being embedded in the triceps muscle, and under the arcade of Struthers, when present. The ulnar nerve becomes once again mobile just proximal to the postcondylar groove of the elbow.

- ♦ In many individuals, there is a C7 contribution to the ulnar nerve, which originates from the lateral cord. This neural communication within the brachial plexus has been labeled *the lateral root of the ulnar nerve.*
- ♦ In a minority of people the antebrachial cutaneous nerve, or even the more proximal medial brachial cutaneous nerve, can originate directly from the ulnar nerve.

2.1.2 The Elbow

After emerging from the medial head of the triceps in the lower arm, the ulnar nerve enters the postcondylar groove. This groove is a curvilinear bony canal between the medial epicondyle of the humerus (lying anterior and medial) and the olecranon of the ulna (posterior and lateral). Within this groove the ulnar nerve is most vulnerable to external trauma. After passing distal to the elbow, the ulnar nerve once again passes below a protective muscle, this time under the flexor carpi ulnaris.

The region just beyond the bony postcondylar groove is the *cubital tunnel.* It has two segments (▶ Fig. 2.4): The first is where the nerve passes under the aponeurosis that connects the two proximal tendons of the flexor carpi ulnaris. Although variable, this aponeurosis can extend proximally, connecting the medial epicondyle to the olecranon. Therefore, it may in fact cover the bony postcondylar groove. The second segment is where the ulnar nerve passes between and under the two muscular heads of the flexor carpi ulnaris. The aponeurosis between the two heads of the flexor carpi ulnaris can be very thick in approximately 75% of the population; in which case it is called the *Osborne band.* As will be discussed, the Osborne band has been implicated in ulnar nerve compression.

Dynamic changes in elbow anatomy are important. As the elbow flexes, the aponeurosis of the flexor carpi ulnaris becomes tense, potentially compressing the ulnar nerve underneath (▶ Fig. 2.5). Furthermore, when the flexor carpi ulnaris muscle contracts, the ulnar nerve may also be compressed under

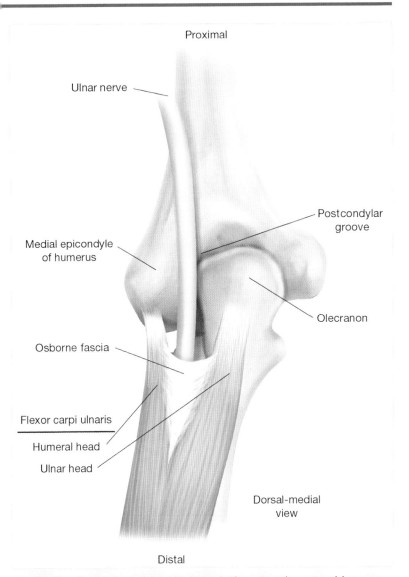

Proximal

Ulnar nerve

Postcondylar
groove

Medial epicondyle
of humerus

Olecranon

Osborne fascia

Flexor carpi ulnaris

Humeral head

Ulnar head

Dorsal-medial
view

Distal

Fig. 2.4 The elbow region and the cubital tunnel. After exiting the postcondylar groove, the ulnar nerve travels through the cubital tunnel. In approximately 75% of the population, the superficial aponeurosis between the two heads of the flexor carpi ulnaris is very thick and is called the Osborne band or fascia.

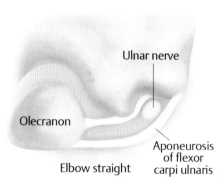

Olecranon

Ulnar nerve

Aponeurosis
of flexor
carpi ulnaris

Elbow straight

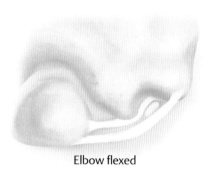

Elbow flexed

Fig. 2.5 The cubital tunnel volume decreases with elbow flexion. Furthermore, contraction of the flexor carpi ulnaris causes the submuscular portion of the cubital tunnel to also constrict (not shown). This is why simultaneous elbow flexion and wrist flexion in an ulnar direction can precipitate symptoms of ulnar entrapment at the elbow.

the second, more distal, portion of the cubital tunnel. This is partly why simultaneous elbow flexion and wrist flexion in an ulnar direction can precipitate symptoms of ulnar entrapment at the elbow.

♦ The amount of aponeurosis covering the postcondylar groove, as well as the space between the two heads of the flexor carpi ulnaris, is variable. In fact, some patients may not have this covering at all, allowing the ulnar nerve to slip, or "snap" over the medial epicondyle during forearm flexion.

♦ The anconeus epitrochlearis muscle is present in approximately 10% of the population. This muscle spans from the medial epicondyle to the olecranon and is a potential cause of ulnar nerve irritation.

2.1.3 The Forearm

After passing deep to the two proximal heads of the flexor carpi ulnaris, the ulnar nerve continues down the forearm under this muscle and above the flexor digitorum profundus. The ulnar nerve usually provides only one major branch to the flexor digitorum profundus, which arises after the branches destined for the flexor carpi ulnaris have already exited. The ulnar nerve passes directly from the medial epicondyle to the pisiform bone in the wrist. In the distal third of the forearm, the ulnar nerve is not covered by muscle; it lies between the flexor carpi ulnaris tendon medially and the flexor digitorum superficialis tendon laterally. The ulnar artery, a branch of the brachial artery in the antecubital fossa, gradually makes its way medially to pair up with the ulnar nerve proximal to the wrist. Once together, these two structures enter the hand, with the artery lateral to the nerve.

Two sensory branches originate from the ulnar nerve in the distal half of the forearm. The first is the *dorsal ulnar cutaneous nerve,* which arises approximately 5 to 10 cm proximal to the wrist crease off the dorsomedial aspect of the ulnar nerve. This branch travels to the dorsum of the distal forearm between the ulna and the tendon of the flexor carpi ulnaris. Once on the dorsal surface, it pierces the antebrachial fascia and becomes subcutaneous a few centimeters proximal to the wrist. The second sensory branch from the ulnar nerve is the *palmar ulnar cutaneous nerve,* which is a mirror image of the palmar cutaneous branch of the median nerve. The palmar ulnar cutaneous nerve branches from the volar-lateral surface of the ulnar nerve approximately 5 to 10 cm proximal to the wrist. It runs adherent to the ulnar nerve for a few centimeters then enters the subcutaneous space proximal to the distal wrist crease and arborizes over the hypothenar eminence.

♦ **Although the dorsal ulnar cutaneous nerve usually originates proximal to the palmar ulnar cutaneous nerve, in certain people the reverse may be true. Alternatively, the dorsal ulnar cutaneous nerve may actually branch from the superficial sensory radial nerve.**

♦ **Communication, or cross talk, between the ulnar nerve and the anterior interosseous nerve via the Martin-Gruber anastomosis may occur in the forearm (see Chapter 1, Median Nerve).**

2.1.4 The Wrist/Hand

In the following discussion, *medial* refers to the hypothenar margin of the hand, and *lateral* refers to the thenar aspect of the hand. The ulnar nerve and artery enter the hand via the Guyon's tunnel (▶ Fig. 2.6). Although the Guyon's tunnel has one proximal entrance, it has two distal exits, one going deeper into the hand and the other remaining superficial. Upon entering this tunnel, the following structures are encountered. First, there is a large protuberance along the medial tunnel wall: the pisiform bone. There is another protuberance, now on the distal lateral side: the hook of the hamate. At the end of the tunnel, there is a fork. The lateral pathway dives deep and almost immediately takes a sharp lateral bend. The medial pathway, however, continues in the same plane

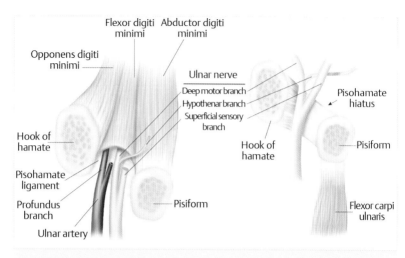

Fig. 2.6 The ulnar nerve at the wrist. The ulnar nerve and artery enter the hand via the Guyon's tunnel. Although the Guyon's tunnel has one proximal entrance, it has two distal exits, one going deeper into the hand and the other remaining superficial.

as the more proximal tunnel. In reviewing the boundaries of the Guyon's tunnel, one needs to consider its proximal and distal segments separately.

For the proximal half of the Guyon's tunnel, the floor is the transverse carpal ligament, and the roof is the superficial palmar carpal ligament (► Fig. 2.7). The small palmaris brevis muscle also runs in the proximal roof of the Guyon's tunnel. By reflecting deeper laterally, the superficial palmar carpal ligament fuses with the transverse carpal ligament below, forming the lateral wall of the Guyon's tunnel. However, the superficial palmar carpal ligament is the lateral wall for the proximal portion of the tunnel only. The flexor carpi ulnaris tendon and the more distal pisiform bone (first bump in the wall described earlier) form the proximal, medial wall of the tunnel.

In the distal half of the tunnel, the lateral wall is formed by the hook of the hamate (second bump in the wall described previously), whereas the shorter medial wall is formed by the pisiform bone. The distal floor is formed initially by the pisohamate ligament, then by the pisometacarpal ligament. The ulnar nerve passes superficial to both of these ligaments. The distal roof of the Guyon's tunnel continues to be formed by the superficial palmar carpal ligament. However, a muscular arch from the pisiform bone to the hook of the hamate forms the roof of the deeper, distal branch tunnel. This muscular arch is mainly from the flexor digiti minimi. Entrance to this deeper branch tunnel has been termed the *pisohamate hiatus.*

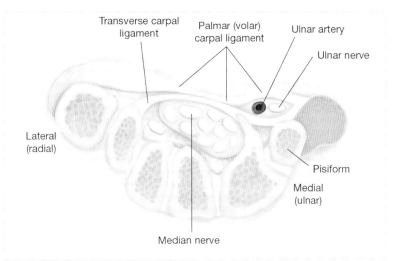

Fig. 2.7 Proximal cross section of the Guyon's tunnel. In the proximal half of the Guyon's tunnel, the floor is the transverse carpal ligament, whereas the roof is the superficial palmar carpal ligament. Reflecting deeper on the lateral margin of the Guyon's tunnel, the superficial palmar carpal ligament forms the lateral wall by fusing with the transverse carpal ligament.

The ulnar nerve bifurcates into a deep motor branch and a superficial sensory branch in the distal Guyon's tunnel. As their names imply, the superficial branch courses through the medial, more superficial tunnel with the ulnar artery, whereas the deep branch goes under the arch created by the flexor digiti minimi with a profunda or deep arterial branch. Prior to this arch, the deep branch of the ulnar nerve yields a small side branch that innervates the hypothenar muscles. Once passing through the Guyon's tunnel into the hand, the deep motor branch curves lateral toward the midline of the hand, remaining deep to the flexor tendons of the fingers. The superficial branch splits into digital nerves destined for the fourth and fifth digits.

♦ Occasionally, there may be early branching of the ulnar nerve with an anomalous course. For example, the ulnar nerve may branch proximal to the pisiform bone, with the superficial sensory branch communicating some, or all, of its sensory fibers to the palmar ulnar cutaneous nerve. A second variation occurs when the deep motor branch bifurcates prior to entering the pisohamate hiatus, with a portion of this nerve entering the carpal tunnel lateral to the hook of the hamate, only to rejoin the usual deep ulnar branch in the palm.

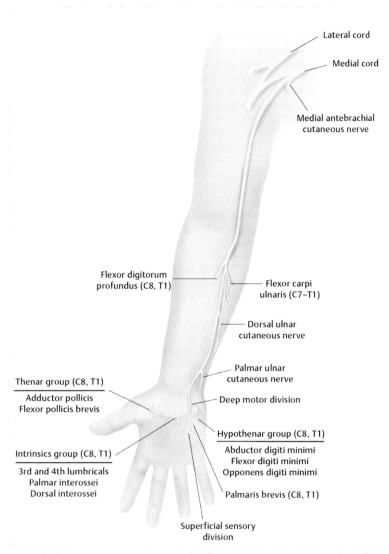

Lateral cord

Medial cord

Medial antebrachial
cutaneous nerve

Flexor digitorum
profundus (C8, T1)

Flexor carpi
ulnaris (C7–T1)

Dorsal ulnar
cutaneous nerve

Palmar ulnar
cutaneous nerve

Thenar group (C8, T1)

Adductor pollicis
Flexor pollicis brevis

Deep motor division

Hypothenar group (C8, T1)

Abductor digiti minimi
Flexor digiti minimi
Opponens digiti minimi

Intrinsics group (C8, T1)

3rd and 4th lumbricals
Palmar interossei
Dorsal interossei

Palmaris brevis (C8, T1)

Superficial sensory
division

Fig. 2.8 Ulnar nerve motor innervation. The ulnar nerve innervates no muscles in the upper arm, yet it is responsible for many fine, coordinated finger movements.

2.2 Motor Innervation and Testing

The ulnar nerve is predominantly responsible for fine hand and finger movements (► Fig. 2.8). The muscles innervated by the ulnar nerve may be grouped as follows: forearm group (two muscles), hypothenar group (four muscles), hand intrinsic muscles (three *groups* of muscles), and the thenar group (two muscles). The ulnar nerve innervates no muscles in the upper arm.

2.2.1 Forearm Group

The first muscle innervated by the ulnar nerve is the *flexor carpi ulnaris* (C7–T1). Branches to this muscle originate in the cubital tunnel, or just distal to it. Testing this muscle is a two-step process. First, while the patient abducts the fifth digit, observe and palpate the flexor carpi ulnaris tendon just proximal to the wrist (► Fig. 2.9). The flexor carpi ulnaris contracts to stabilize the pisiform so that the abductor digiti minimi may abduct the fifth digit. Next, have the patient flex the wrist against resistance in an ulnar direction (► Fig. 2.10), which is the primary action of this muscle.

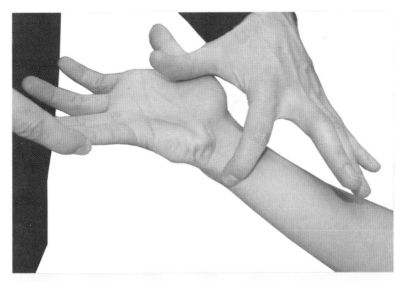

Fig. 2.9 Flexor carpi ulnaris (C7, T1) assessment, stabilizing the pisiform: While the patient abducts the ipsilateral fifth digit, observe and palpate the flexor carpi ulnaris tendon just proximal to the wrist. The flexor carpi ulnaris contracts to stabilize the pisiform so that the abductor digiti minimi may function.

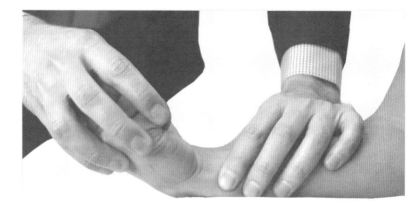

Fig. 2.10 Flexor carpi ulnaris (C7, T1) assessment, wrist flexion: Have the patient flex the wrist against resistance in an ulnar direction, which is the primary action of this muscle.

The second muscle innervated by the ulnar nerve in the forearm is the *flexor digitorum profundus* (C8, T1) to the fourth and fifth digits. Branches to this muscle originate when the ulnar nerve is between the flexor digitorum profundus and the flexor carpi ulnaris in the proximal forearm. This muscle is tested in the same fashion as for its median innervated half, except one uses the fifth digit: immobilize the proximal interphalangeal joint while the patient flexes the distal interphalangeal joint (▶ Fig. 2.11).

- In 5% of patients, branches to the flexor carpi ulnaris originate proximal to the elbow.
- Although the median nerve's anterior interosseous branch may occasionally control distal interphalangeal joint flexion of the ring finger (in addition to the index and long fingers), the ulnar nerve always controls this movement in the fifth digit.

2.2.2 Hypothenar Group

The ulnar nerve bifurcates into two divisions within the Guyon's tunnel: the superficial sensory and the deep motor. The superficial sensory division innervates only one, often forgotten, muscle, the *palmaris brevis* (C8, T1). The small branch that innervates this muscle usually originates from the sensory division as it leaves the distal end of the Guyon's tunnel. The palmaris brevis is located in the roof of the Guyon's tunnel, and, when contracted, corrugates the hypothenar skin. This deepens the hollow of the hand, possibly aiding in grasp. To test

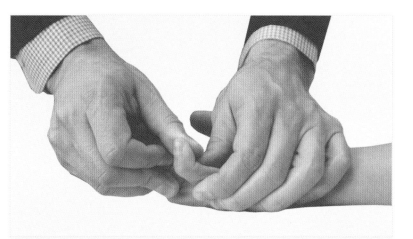

Fig. 2.11 Flexor digitorum profundus (C8, T1) assessment: This muscle is tested in the same fashion as its median innervated half, except, to evaluate the ulnar nerve contribution, one uses the fifth digit. To test, immobilize the proximal interphalangeal joint while the patient flexes the distal interphalangeal joint against resistance.

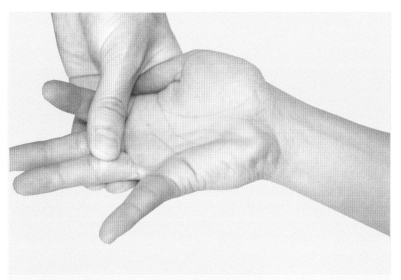

Fig. 2.12 Palmaris brevis (C8, T1) assessment: Test this muscle by having the patient forcibly abduct the fifth digit and then "contract" the hypothenar eminence. Skin corrugation should occur.

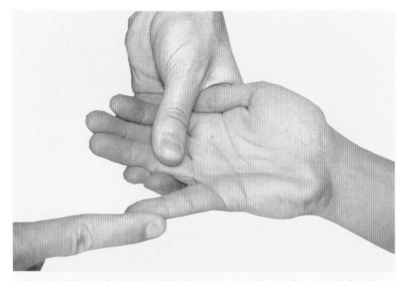

Fig. 2.13 Abductor digiti minimi (C8, T1) assessment: This muscle is tested when the patient abducts the fifth digit against resistance. One should keep in mind that this muscle is delicate, and the patient's resistance is easily overcome by the examiner.

this muscle, have the patient forcibly abduct the fifth digit and "contract" the hypothenar eminence. Skin corrugation should occur (▶ Fig. 2.12).

The deep motor division gives a small motor branch to the hypothenar eminence just before diving into the pisohamate hiatus. This branch innervates the three muscles of the hypothenar eminence: the abductor digiti minimi, the flexor digiti minimi, and the opponens digiti minimi. The *abductor digiti minimi* (C8, T1) is tested when the patient abducts the fifth digit against resistance (▶ Fig. 2.13). One should keep in mind that this muscle is delicate, with even normal strength being easily overcome by the examiner. The *flexor digiti minimi* (C8, T1) may be assessed by immobilizing the interphalangeal joints of the fifth digit and instructing the patient to flex the metacarpal–phalangeal joint against resistance (▶ Fig. 2.14). One cannot isolate this muscle's function because flexion of the fifth digit's metacarpal–phalangeal joint is performed not only by the flexor digiti minimi but also by the fourth lumbrical and the interossei. Next, test the *opponens digiti minimi* (C8, T1) by having the patient hold the volar pads of the distal thumb and fifth digit together. While the patient maintains this position, try to force the distal fifth metacarpal away from the thumb (▶ Fig. 2.15). Hypothenar wasting may be evident with chronic denervation of these muscles.

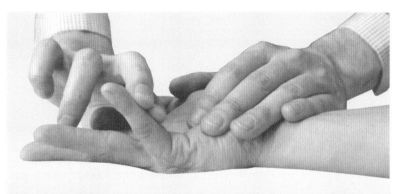

Fig. 2.14 Flexor digiti minimi (C8, T1) assessment: This muscle is tested by immobilizing the interphalangeal joints of the fifth digit and having the patient flex the metacarpal–phalangeal (knuckle) joint against resistance. One cannot isolate this muscle's function because flexion of the fifth digit's metacarpal–phalangeal joint is also performed by the fourth lumbrical and interossei.

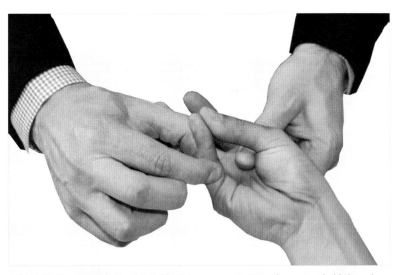

Fig. 2.15 Opponens digiti minimi (C8, T1) assessment: Have the patient hold the volar pads of the distal thumb and fifth digit together. While the patient maintains this position, try to force the distal fifth metacarpal away from the thumb.

2.2.3 Hand Intrinsic Muscles

The small and deeply situated hand intrinsic muscles may be placed into three groups: lumbricals, palmar interossei, and dorsal interossei. The lumbricals help flex the metacarpal–phalangeal joints and extend the proximal inter-phalangeal joints when the metacarpal–phalangeal joints are immobilized in a hyperextended position. The dorsal interossei abduct or spread the fingers. The palmar interossei adduct or close the fingers; they also assist the lumbricals in flexing the metacarpal–phalangeal joints. The deep branch of the ulnar nerve innervates the third and fourth lumbricals (to the fourth and fifth digits), as well as all of the palmar and dorsal interossei muscles.

To test the *third and fourth lumbricals* (C8, T1), immobilize the metacarpal–phalangeal joints of these two fingers in hyperextension and then test exten-sion of the proximal interphalangeal joints against resistance (▶ Fig. 2.16). A simple way to test the interossei is to concentrate on the index finger. On a flat surface have the patient both abduct (*first dorsal interosseus* [C8, T1]) (▶ Fig. 2.17) or adduct (*second palmar interosseous* [C8, T1]) (▶ Fig. 2.18) the index finger against resistance. Contraction of the first dorsal interosseous muscle can be observed and palpated on the dorsum of the hand. When dorsal interossei muscle wasting is present, the extensor tendons on the dorsum of the hand appear more prominent when compared with the normal hand.

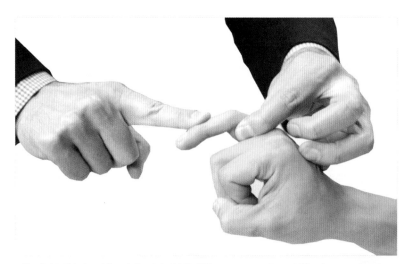

Fig. 2.16 Third and fourth lumbrical (C8, T1) assessment: Immobilize the metacarpal–phalangeal joints of these two fingers in hyperextension and then test extension of the proximal interphalangeal joints against resistance.

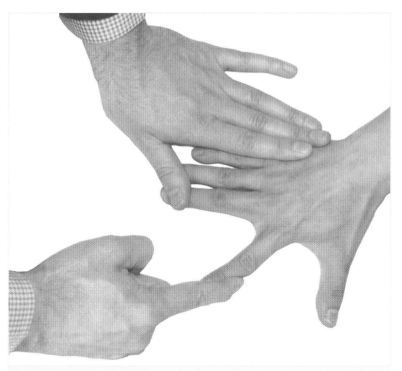

Fig. 2.17 First dorsal interosseous (C8, T1) assessment: On a flat surface, the patient abducts the index finger against resistance. Contraction and/or atrophy of the first dorsal interosseous muscle can be observed and palpated on the dorsum of the hand.

Another way to assess the palmar interossei is by having the patient maintain the extended fingers together when you attempt to pass a digit between them.

♦ **The long finger flexors (flexor digitorum superficialis and flexor digitorum profundus) can substitute for digit adduction when the fingers are actively flexed. The finger extensors, in corollary, can help abduct the digits when the fingers are actively extended. To eliminate these substitutions and isolate the interossei, the fingers should be in extension at the metacarpal–phalangeal joints when assessed.**

2.2.4 Thenar Group

The ulnar nerve innervates two muscles of the median nerve–dominated thenar eminence. The first is the *adductor pollicis* (C8, T1). Test this muscle by

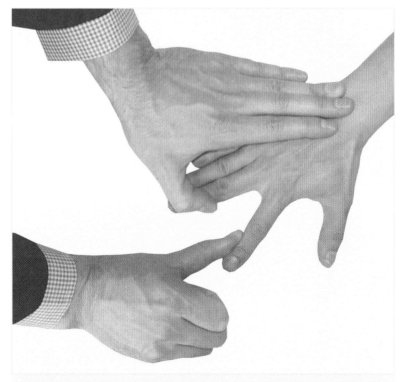

Fig. 2.18 Second palmar interosseous (C8, T1) assessment: On a flat surface, the patient adducts the index finger against resistance. Alternatively, the patient can be instructed to keep the extended fingers together as you attempt to pass a digit between them (not shown).

having the patient adduct the straightened thumb along a plane parallel to the palm (▶ Fig. 2.19). Try to separate the thumb from the lateral border of the palm. Alternatively, you may place your index finger between the patient's thumb and lateral palm, applying resistance as the thumb is adducted. Because of its large size, atrophy of this muscle alone may cause thenar wasting.

The second muscle is the deep head of the *flexor pollicis brevis* (C8, T1), with its superficial head being innervated by the median nerve. Although not a very useful muscle to test because of its dual innervation, some weakness compared with the other side may be seen with ulnar lesions. To test this muscle, the patient flexes the thumb's metacarpal–phalangeal joint while the inter-phalangeal joint is maintained in extension to minimize substitution by the flexor pollicis longus (▶ Fig. 2.20).

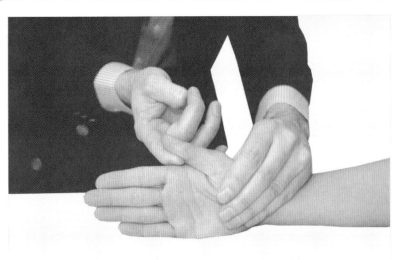

Fig. 2.19 Adductor pollicis (C8, T1) assessment: Test this muscle by having the patient adduct a straightened thumb in the plane parallel to the palm. Try to separate the thumb from the lateral border of the palm. Alternatively, you may place your index finger between the thumb and lateral palm, applying resistance as the thumb is adducted (shown).

2.2.5 Martin-Gruber and Riche-Cannieu Anastomoses

As mentioned in Chapter 1, the median and ulnar nerves may communicate with each other in the forearm via the anterior interosseus nerve (Martin-Gruber anastomosis). A second communication may occur in the deep palm between the thenar motor branch of the median nerve and the deep motor division of the ulnar nerve (Riche-Cannieu anastomosis). Minor and major shifts in motor innervation of the hand may occur through these two potential routes of communication.

The Riche-Cannieu anastomosis, although anatomically present in the majority of patients, does not always communicate axons that shift innervation between the median and ulnar nerves. However, when a transfer does occur, this connection either returns thenar innervation that was transferred to the ulnar nerve in the forearm via the Martin-Gruber anastomosis, or it acts as a conduit for the median nerve to innervate all the lumbricals, not only the first two. An important principle to remember is that, when strange patterns of deficits occur following median or ulnar nerve injury, one should consider these potential communications when deciding if an injury is complete or incomplete.

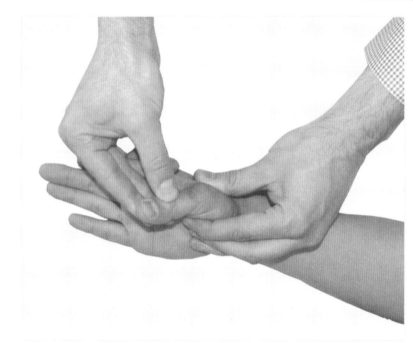

Fig. 2.20 Flexor pollicis brevis (C8, T1) assessment: Although not a useful muscle to test because of its dual innervation (median and ulnar nerves), some weakness compared with the other side may be present with ulnar lesions. To test this muscle, the patient flexes the thumb's metacarpal–phalangeal joint while the interphalangeal joint is maintained in extension to minimize substitution by the flexor pollicis longus muscle.

2.3 Sensory Innervation

Aside from the medial brachial and antebrachial cutaneous nerves, which originate from the medial cord (described previously), the ulnar nerve proper has three sensory branches. These branches provide sensory innervation to the medial third of the hand (▶ Fig. 2.21).

The *dorsal ulnar cutaneous nerve* pierces the antebrachial fascia just proximal to the dorsomedial wrist. It crosses the wrist and ramifies to innervate the dorsomedial third of the hand. It also innervates the dorsum of the fifth and the medial half of the fourth digits. However, the skin under and surrounding the fingernail is innervated by the superficial sensory division of the ulnar nerve, whose branches arise from the volar surface of the hand. Sensory testing for the dorsal ulnar cutaneous nerve should take place on the dorsal surface of the medial third of the hand.

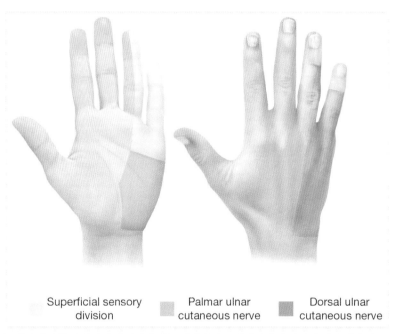

| Superficial sensory division | Palmar ulnar cutaneous nerve | Dorsal ulnar cutaneous nerve |

Fig. 2.21 Ulnar nerve sensory territory. The ulnar nerve has three sensory branches. These branches provide sensory innervation to the medial third of the hand.

The *palmar ulnar cutaneous nerve* enters the subcutaneous space of the hypothenar eminence and provides sensory innervation to this area. This nerve innervates the whole medial third of the palm. However, because of sensory territory variations, the best area to test this nerve's function is on the hypothenar eminence.

The *superficial sensory division* of the ulnar nerve, aside from innervating the palmaris brevis muscle, remains a pure sensory nerve. It carries sensation from the volar surface of the fifth and the medial half of the fourth digits, including the dorsal aspect of the distal phalanges (fingernails). The digital nerves carry sensation from the fingers to the superficial sensory division. The optimal area to test autonomous sensation for this nerve is on the volar aspect of the fifth digit.

♦ There may be frequent variation in sensory territories between these three ulnar branches. For example, the palmar ulnar cutaneous nerve may cover only the proximal hypothenar eminence, with the superficial sensory division covering the remaining medial, volar surface of the palm. Another common variation is for the median nerve (more common) or ulnar nerve, to carry all the sensory fibers from the fourth digit.

49

2.4 Clinical Findings and Syndromes

In contrast to the median nerve, where entrapment usually occurs at the wrist and rarely in the proximal forearm/elbow, for the ulnar nerve the opposite is true: it is often compressed at the elbow and rarely at the wrist.

2.4.1 The Arm

Complete Palsy

Ulnar nerve palsies in the upper arm are usually traumatic, including gunshot wounds, lacerations, and blunt injuries. Because of their close proximity, the median nerve and brachial artery may sustain concomitant injury. As with the median nerve, the ulnar nerve may be compressed by a crutch or by the arm hanging over a chair *(Saturday night palsy)*.

Considering the loss of fine coordinated hand movements, a complete ulnar nerve lesion is quite devastating. To begin, a severe ulnar lesion causes loss of sensation in the hypothenar eminence (palmar ulnar cutaneous branch), the volar surface of the fifth and half of the fourth digits (superficial sensory division), and the dorsomedial third of the hand and fingers (dorsal ulnar cutaneous nerve). If sensory abnormalities extend more than 2 cm proximal to the wrist crease one should consider involvement of the medial antebrachial cutaneous nerve, and therefore the medial cord of the brachial plexus or C8/T1 nerve roots. With complete ulnar nerve palsies, wrist flexion in an ulnar direction is absent. The distal phalanges of the fourth and especially the fifth digits will not flex secondary to flexor digitorum profundus weakness. Marked hand intrinsic weakness occurs, with residual function provided only by the median nerve–innervated thenar muscles. Muscle wasting is often present, including the hypothenar eminence, dorsal interosseous muscles, and even the thenar eminence secondary to wasting of the large adductor pollicis. There is loss of finger abduction and adduction from paralysis of the dorsal and palmar interossei, respectively. However, as mentioned earlier, some finger abduction or adduction can still occur because of substitution by the long finger flexors and extensors.

Ulnar claw hand is most prominent when the patient is opening the hand: there is hyperextension at the metacarpal–phalangeal joints in the fourth and especially the fifth digits, along with partial flexion of both interphalangeal joints in these two fingers (▶ Fig. 2.22). Ulnar claw hand results from a loss of function in the third and fourth lumbricals, along with paralysis of the interossei and flexor digit minimi, which causes flexion weakness at the metacarpal–phalangeal joints. The extensor digitorum communis (radial nerve) becomes unopposed, thereby placing these two metacarpal–phalangeal joints in hyperextension. Despite paralysis of the flexor digitorum profundus in these two

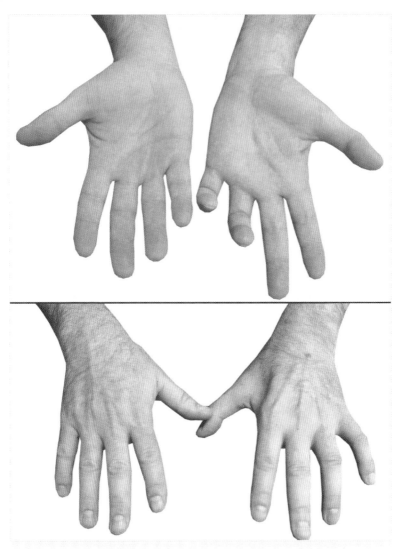

Fig. 2.22 Ulnar claw hand (patient's left). There is hyperextension of the metacarpal–phalangeal joints in the fourth and especially the fifth digits. Both interphalangeal joints are also partially flexed in these two fingers. Atrophy of the first dorsal interosseous muscle is evident on the dorsal view (bottom). The patient's normal right hand is shown for comparison.

digits, its tendons still have tension. This is because of the hyperextension mentioned earlier, as well as from residual tone in this muscle from its median nerve–innervated portion. Furthermore, when a severe or complete ulnar nerve lesion occurs distal to the flexor digitorum profundus (i.e., a lesion that spares this muscle), the degree of claw hand is worse because even more unopposed distal finger flexion occurs. Without proper physical therapy, ulnar claw hand may become permanent from muscle contractures.

When the fifth digit is slightly more abducted compared with the normal hand it is referred to as the *Wartenberg sign*. This occurs because the third palmar interosseous muscle, which adducts the fifth digit, is paralyzed; unopposed action of the extensor digiti minimi and extensor digitorum communis of the radial nerve causes the finger to rest in a slightly more abducted position.

A *Froment paper sign* can be elicited when the patient is asked to pull apart a piece of paper held between the complete volar surface of each straightened thumb and closed fist (▶ Fig. 2.23). In the affected hand, the adductor pollicis is weak, and thumb adduction does not occur. Instead, the interphalangeal joint of the affected thumb flexes to hold the paper through contraction of the flexor pollicis longus (median innervated).

Arcade of Struthers

Once it has pierced the intermuscular septum about halfway down the arm, the ulnar nerve is enveloped by the medial head of the triceps. In approximately 50% of the population, an arcade of fascia, the arcade of Struthers, extends over the ulnar nerve from the intermuscular septum to the superficial surface of the medial head of the triceps. This arcade is a few centimeters in length and occurs approximately 8 cm proximal to the elbow.

The arcade of Struthers, in fact, does not cause primary ulnar nerve compression. Instead, its presence may predispose some ulnar nerve transpositions at the elbow to failure; the arcade of Struthers, when present and not transected during the original transposition surgery, may tether the relocated ulnar nerve, which leads to compression and continued symptoms (▶ Fig. 2.24).

2.4.2 The Elbow

Olecranon Notch

Compression of the ulnar nerve at the elbow is a common entrapment, second only to carpal tunnel syndrome (▶ Fig. 2.25). It usually presents with sensory changes in the fifth and fourth digits, including hyperesthesia, hypesthesia, and paresthesias. At first, these symptoms are intermittent, often induced by prolonged forearm flexion or direct compression of the ulnar nerve in the

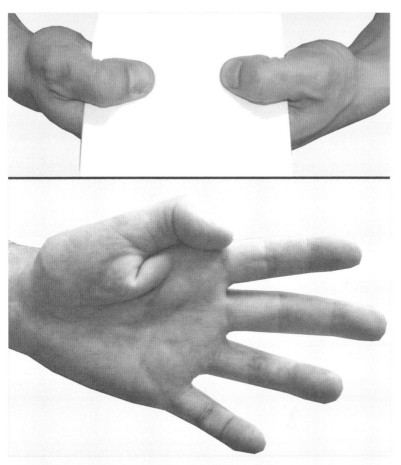

Fig. 2.23 The Froment paper sign. When the adductor pollicis is weak, thumb adduction does not occur. Instead, contraction of the flexor pollicis longus muscle substitutes for this movement by flexing the interphalangeal joint of the thumb. The upper photograph illustrates a bilateral Froment paper sign when a subject attempts to pull apart a piece of paper. The lower figure reveals a Froment paper sign when the patient is instructed to hold a straightened thumb against the lateral margin of the hand.

postcondylar grove. One should inquire about repetitive actions and a history of trauma. These sensory symptoms can occur at night if, during sleep, the arm is flexed or the elbow lies on a hard surface when the forearm is extended and supinated, thus exposing the ulnar nerve to compression. Although not as common as with carpal tunnel syndrome, symptoms from ulnar nerve

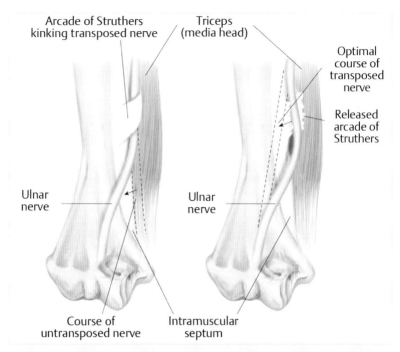

Fig. 2.24 Arcade of Struthers compressing a transposed ulnar nerve. When this fascial arcade is present and not transected during the original transposition surgery, then a medially transposed nerve at the elbow may become tethered at the arcade of Struthers, leading to a new area of compression and continued symptoms.

compression at the elbow can wake the patient up at night. Abnormal light touch and vibration sense may be evident on examination. Provocative maneuvers, like flexing the forearm for a minute, may precipitate symptoms. The patient should also repetitively flex the elbow while the ulnar nerve is palpated in the postcondylar groove to rule out "snapping" or dislocation of either the ulnar nerve or medial triceps tendon, both of which can cause ulnar nerve irritation at the elbow. One must keep in mind, however, that the majority of patients with prolapsing ulnar nerves are asymptomatic.

As nerve damage progresses, patients usually report numbness that is more persistent. They report pain in the postcondylar region, often radiating down the medial forearm to the hand. A Tinel sign at the postcondylar groove may be present. With more nerve damage, patients begin to have weakness in the ulnar-innervated hand intrinsic muscles. They may report clumsiness with fine hand movements, like buttoning buttons or using a pen. With moderate to

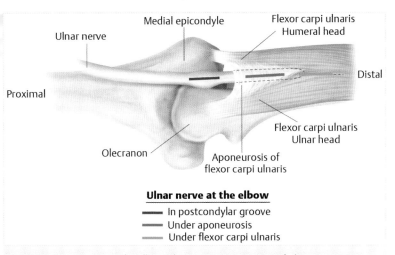

Medial epicondyle

Flexor carpi ulnaris
Humeral head

Ulnar nerve

Distal

Proximal

Flexor carpi ulnaris
Ulnar head

Olecranon

Aponeurosis of
flexor carpi ulnaris

Ulnar nerve at the elbow

━━━ In postcondylar groove
━━━ Under aponeurosis
━━━ Under flexor carpi ulnaris

Fig. 2.25 Compression at the elbow. The most common point of ulnar nerve injury, as evidenced by intraoperative nerve action potential recordings, is at the postcondylar groove just proximal to its covering aponeurosis. Other points of possible ulnar nerve entrapment at the elbow are between the two heads of the flexor carpi ulnaris (cubital tunnel syndrome), and the Osborne fascia, when present.

severe damage, two-point discrimination is also affected. To ascertain subtle hand intrinsic weakness, one can observe the following finger movements (compared with the normal hand): rapid thumb to fingertip touching (observe slowing and lack of precision), synchronous digit flexion and extension (look for early claw hand), and if available, power grip testing (usually decreased up to 80% with ulnar palsies).

With more severe and chronic compression, persistent numbness, hand intrinsic weakness, ulnar nerve tenderness at the elbow, and muscular atrophy may be present. When atrophy occurs, it is most readily noted at the hypothenar eminence and first dorsal interosseous muscle. Median nerve–innervated hand intrinsics (e.g., abductor pollicis brevis) should be normal, or else a C8/T1 spinal nerve/lower trunk/medial cord lesion may be present (e.g., neurogenic thoracic outlet syndrome). Ulnar claw hand, the Wartenberg sign, and the Froment paper sign are all usually present in severe, chronic cases. Despite branches to the flexor carpi ulnaris often originating from the ulnar nerve distal to the postcondylar groove, weakness of this muscle in cubital tunnel syndrome is rare. This has been attributed to the fact that the sensory and hand intrinsic fibers in the ulnar nerve at the elbow are more superficial, and, perhaps, more prone to irritation. If flexor carpi ulnaris weakness is present or occurs early, a lesion more proximal to the postcondylar groove should be considered.

The most common point of ulnar nerve damage, as evidenced by intra-operative nerve action potential recordings, is at the postcondylar groove just proximal to its covering aponeurosis. Other points of possible ulnar nerve entrapment at the elbow include between the two heads of the flexor carpi ulnaris (cubital tunnel syndrome) and by the Osborne fascia, when present.

♦ Tardive ulnar palsy is late-onset ulnar nerve compression at the elbow following an elbow fracture years earlier. In these patients, the fracture causes a capitus valgus deformity at the elbow (the forearm is angled laterally when the elbow is extended). This anatomical situation increases tension on the medially located ulnar nerve (by increasing the distance it must travel), thereby predisposing it to compression at the elbow.

♦ The anconeus muscle, which runs between the medial epicondyle and the olecranon in some patients, may also cause ulnar nerve entrapment at the elbow.

♦ The most frequent operative positioning injury affects the ulnar nerve at the elbow.

2.4.3 The Forearm

Flexor–Pronator Fascia

Although exceedingly rare, the ulnar nerve may be irritated by a thickened flexor–pronator fascia. Compression by this structure would occur in the proximal to midforearm (approximately 5 cm distal to the medial epicondyle), where the ulnar nerve passes between the flexor carpi ulnaris and the flexor digitorum profundus. Fascia between these muscles may be excessively thick, thereby predisposing the nerve to compression. Although a clear syndrome has not been reported, repetitive forearm pronation and wrist flexion are thought to be associated with this form of compression.

The Dorsal Ulnar Cutaneous Nerve

Occasionally, the dorsal ulnar cutaneous branch may be compressed or transected as it leaves the ulnar nerve and passes to the dorsum of the wrist between the flexor carpi ulnaris tendon and the ulna. Ulnar fractures or repairs, lacerations, or blunt trauma may involve this nerve. Patients present with numbness or hypesthesia in the dorsomedial third of the hand. With some lesions, a Tinel sign can be elicited when tapping on the medial border of the ulna a few centimeters proximal to the wrist.

2.4.4 The Wrist

Guyon's Tunnel

Ulnar nerve compression at the wrist is rare. Nonetheless, based on the ulnar nerve's branching pattern in the Guyon's tunnel, three zones of compression have been described: zone 1, compression of the ulnar nerve prior to its division within the Guyon's tunnel; zone 2, compression of only the deep motor division; and zone 3, compression of only the superficial sensory division (▶ Fig. 2.26).

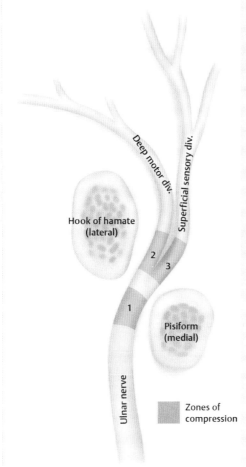

Fig. 2.26 Zones of compression in the Guyon's tunnel. Based on the ulnar nerve's branching pattern in the Guyon's tunnel, three zones of compression have been described: zone 1, compression of the ulnar nerve prior to its division in the Guyon's tunnel (most common); zone 2, compression of only the deep motor branch; and zone 3, compression of only the superficial sensory division (least common).

Deep motor div.

Superficial sensory div.

Hook of hamate (lateral)

2

3

1

Pisiform (medial)

Ulnar nerve

Zones of compression

Zone 1 lesions affect the ulnar nerve before it divides. The etiology is usually a fracture or ganglion cyst compressing the nerve in the proximal portion of the Guyon's tunnel. Sensory loss occurs on the volar surfaces of the fifth and medial half of the fourth fingers, including the nail beds. Sensation to the hypothenar eminence is commonly spared because the palmar ulnar cutaneous nerve is unaffected. Patients with zone 1 compression can have intrinsic hand muscle weakness, including a claw hand, a Wartenberg sign, and a Froment paper sign. The claw hand can be quite severe because innervation to the flexor digitorum profundus is preserved.

Zone 2 lesions compress only the deep motor branch; therefore, no cutaneous sensory loss is present. The motor deficits are similar to a zone 1 lesion. To confirm that the superficial sensory division is intact, one may check for a *palmaris brevis sign,* which is simply observing the contraction of the palmaris brevis (see **Fig. 2.12**). Innervation of this small muscle is from the proximal superficial sensory division; therefore, if this muscle contracts, one knows that this division is at least partially functioning. Zone 2 lesions are usually caused by ganglion cysts. Occasionally, the hypothenar branch from the deep motor division is affected in isolation, causing only weakness in the hypothenar muscles.

Zone 3 lesions affect only the superficial sensory division and are the least common variety of ulnar entrapment at the wrist. A reliable area to test for sensory loss is on the volar surface of the fifth digit. All motor function is usually spared, and the palmaris brevis sign may be absent (no contraction). A distal ulnar artery thrombosis or aneurysm may be causative.

Ulnar nerve compression at the wrist can also be secondary to direct pressure. This can result from prolonged writing, from using a computer or mouse, and from riding a bicycle. These lesions present with a combination of motor and sensory symptoms and usually respond well to rest and behavior modification.

3 Radial Nerve

3.1 Anatomical Course

3.1.1 The Axilla

Following the thoracodorsal and axillary nerve branches, the posterior cord of the brachial plexus becomes the radial nerve, which is composed of axons from the C5–C8 spinal nerves. In contrast to the anterior location of the median and ulnar nerves, the radial nerve remains posterior to the axillary artery in the axilla.

Entering the upper arm, the radial nerve remains superficial to three sequential muscles and/or tendons, which together constitute the posterior axillobrachial border (from proximal to distal): (1) the subscapularis muscle inserting into the humeral head, (2) the latissimus dorsi muscle inserting into the surgical neck of the humerus, and, shortly thereafter, (3) the teres major muscle also inserting into the surgical neck of the humerus (▶ Fig. 3.1). The radial nerve continues down the upper arm on the anterior surface of the long head of the triceps, a muscle that originates from the lateral scapula in the axilla.

♦ In approximately 10% of the general population the radial nerve also carries fibers from the T1 spinal nerve.

3.1.2 The Axilla to the Spiral Groove

The triceps has three heads—long, medial, and lateral—all of which share a common insertion on the olecranon. These three heads act in unison to extend the forearm. Their names are derived from their respective origins. The *long* head is so named because its course is *long* from its scapular origin, high in the axilla, down to the olecranon. The *medial* head of the triceps originates along the *medial* (and posterior) humeral shaft, is *medial* (and anterior) to the long head of the triceps, and remains *medial* (and posterior) to the humerus. The *lateral* head originates along the *lateral* humeral shaft, remaining *lateral* to both the long head of the triceps and the humerus. The origins of the lateral and medial heads of the triceps run parallel along the humerus in a spiral fashion (▶ Fig. 3.2). These insertions begin posteromedially, then curve posterior and lateral down the humerus. The bare area of bone between the origins of the lateral and medial heads of the triceps is called the *spiral groove.*

After entering the upper arm superficial to the long head of the triceps, the radial nerve immediately dives into a cleft between the long and medial heads of the triceps (▶ Fig. 3.1). The brachial profunda artery runs with the radial nerve in this cleft. Together they course posteriorly and medially toward the

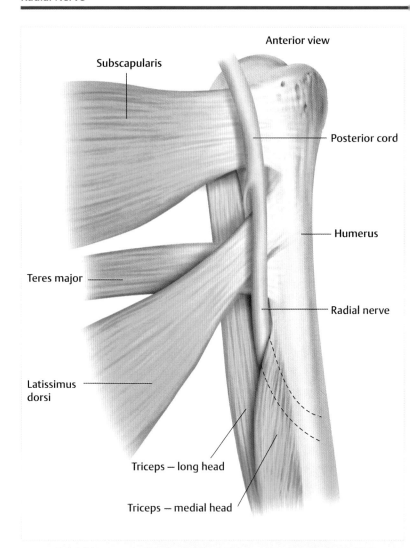

Fig. 3.1 Radial nerve in the distal axilla. The radial nerve lies superficial to three sequential muscles as it exits the axilla (from proximal to distal): the subscapularis inserting into the humeral head; the latissimus dorsi tendon inserting into both the head and the surgical neck of the humerus; and the teres major inserting into the surgical neck of the humerus. The radial nerve enters the arm anterior to the long head of the triceps. It soon dives into a cleft between the long triceps head and the medial triceps head. Within this cleft, the nerve runs toward the spiral groove.

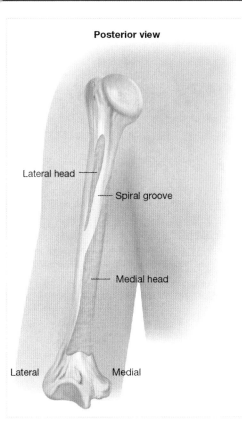

Posterior view

Fig. 3.2 Origin of medial and lateral heads of the triceps on the humerus (posterior view). Their origins run parallel along the humerus in a spiral fashion. This spiral begins posteromedially and curves distally by running posterior, then lateral, along the humerus.

Lateral head

Spiral groove

Medial head

Lateral   Medial

spiral groove. The radial nerve passes down the spiral groove (i.e., posterior and lateral to the humerus) between the origins of the lateral and medial heads of the triceps. It remains in contact with the humerus and is covered by the lateral head of the triceps until it pierces the lateral intermuscular septum, about halfway down the arm, just distal to the deltoid's insertion into the humerus.

3.1.3 The Spiral Groove to the Supinator Muscle

Distal to the spiral groove, the radial nerve enters the flexor compartment by piercing the lateral intermuscular septum. At this location, the radial nerve is immobile and superficial, making it prone to injury. Once in the flexor compartment, from mid-upper arm to antecubital fossa, the radial nerve runs

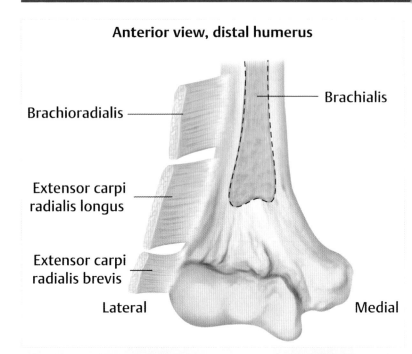

Anterior view, distal humerus

Brachioradialis

Brachialis

Extensor carpi radialis longus

Extensor carpi radialis brevis

Lateral

Medial

Fig. 3.3 Upon entering the flexor compartment at midarm level, the radial nerve runs under three muscles, which sequentially arcade over the nerve. This anatomical arrangement has been referred to as the radial tunnel. The origins of these muscles are depicted.

underneath the following three muscles, which sequentially arcade over the nerve: (1) the brachioradialis, (2) the extensor carpi radialis longus, and (3) the extensor carpi radialis brevis (► Fig. 3.3). This arcade of muscles is referred to as the *radial tunnel*. The last muscle, the extensor carpi radialis brevis, uniquely originates underneath the nerve, but subsequently loops over it; an anatomical arrangement that may predispose the radial nerve to irritation. Along the radial tunnel, the brachialis muscle lies medial and posterior to the radial nerve. The lateral epicondyle of the humerus is posterior.

Distal to the elbow joint, the radial nerve lies on the most proximal portion of the supinator muscle's deep head (see later discussion). Here the radial nerve bifurcates into the posterior interosseous and superficial sensory radial nerves. The location of this bifurcation is variable, being either proximal or distal to the lateral epicondyle.

Allow your right arm to hang at your side in the anatomical position (supinated). Grasp your right forearm with your left hand, just distal to the lateral epicondyle, so that the web space between your thumb and index finger is on the lateral border of the arm with your fingertips pointed in the direction of the elbow joint. Your left hand is the supinator muscle. The supinator muscle originates from the anterior, lateral, and posterior aspects of the radial bone (your palm), and it attaches more proximally to the anterior and lateral portions of the lateral epicondyle of the humerus (thumb tip), as well as to the most superior portion of the ulna's posterior surface (fingertips). As the forearm pronates with an extended elbow, the supinator muscle is stretched as the radius crosses anterior to the ulna. When this extended muscle subsequently contracts, the forearm resupinates.

The supinator has both a deep and a superficial head. If you had two left hands, and you put the second one on top of the first, it would replicate the anatomical relationship between these two heads. The superficial head forms a pocket, into which the posterior interosseous nerve descends. The edge of this pocket can be fibrous and is termed the *arcade of Fröhse.* The superficial sensory radial nerve remains superficial to both heads of the supinator (▶ Fig. 3.4)

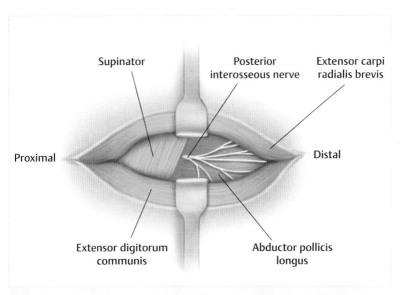

Fig. 3.4 Once emerging from between the two heads of the supinator muscle in the extensor compartment of the dorsal forearm, the posterior interosseous nerve lies deep to the extensor digitorum communis but superficial to the abductor pollicis longus. It ramifies into a large number of unnamed branches, which are often called the cauda equina of the arm.

3.1.4 The Posterior Interosseous Nerve

The posterior interosseous nerve carries no cutaneous sensation; therefore, it is a "pure" motor nerve. It enters the supinator pocket, deep to the arcade of Fröhse. The recurrent radial artery, a branch of the radial artery, enters the supinator pocket with the posterior interosseous nerve. Once between the two heads of the supinator muscle, the posterior interosseous nerve travels laterally around the head of the radius, entering the extensor compartment of the forearm. Sometimes the posterior interosseous nerve may actually lie directly on the radius when the deep head of the supinator muscle is thin or partly absent. After emerging from between the two heads of the supinator muscle in the extensor compartment of the forearm, the posterior interosseous nerve lies deep to the extensor digitorum communis and superficial to the abductor pollicis longus. It then ramifies into a large number of unnamed branches, which are often called the *cauda equina of the forearm* (▶ Fig. 3.5). While remaining underneath the extensor digitorum communis muscle, the posterior interosseous nerve and its branches run in sequence over the abductor pollicis longus, the extensor pollicis longus, and the extensor pollicis brevis (the three radial nerve–innervated thumb muscles). Distally, along the bottom third of the forearm, the remaining branches of the posterior interosseous nerve are quite deep, lying directly on (posterior to) the interosseous membrane. Here, the posterior interosseous artery, a branch of the interosseous communis artery (from the ulnar artery) joins these terminal nerve branches.

3.1.5 The Superficial Sensory Radial Nerve

This terminal branch of the radial nerve remains superficial to the supinator muscle but deep to the brachioradialis muscle. In fact, it remains under the brachioradialis muscle until approximately two thirds of the way down the forearm (▶ Fig. 3.4). The superficial sensory radial nerve also runs adjacent and parallel to the extensor carpi radialis longus muscle. In the lower third of the forearm, this nerve becomes superficial when the brachioradialis and extensor carpi radialis longus form their tendons. Between these tendons on the lateral edge of the radius the superficial sensory radial nerve pierces the antebrachial fascia and becomes subcutaneous. Here the nerve passes to the dorsal aspect of the wrist, branches upon the dorsolateral aspect of the hand, and remains superficial to the extensor retinaculum. The superficial sensory radial nerve usually has four or more terminal sensory branches.

3.2 Motor Innervation and Testing

The radial nerve innervates four groups of muscles: the triceps group (one muscle, three heads), the lateral epicondyle group (four muscles), the posterior

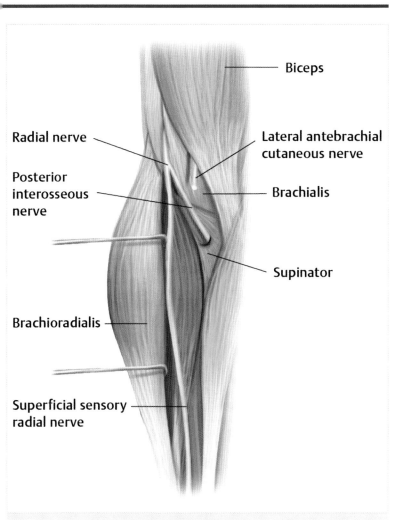

Fig. 3.5 The superficial sensory radial nerve in the distal forearm. This terminal branch of the radial nerve passes distally between the brachioradialis and extensor carpi radialis muscles.

Labels:
- Biceps
- Radial nerve
- Lateral antebrachial cutaneous nerve
- Posterior interosseous nerve
- Brachialis
- Supinator
- Brachioradialis
- Superficial sensory radial nerve

interosseous nerve—superficial group (three muscles), and the posterior inter-osseous nerve—deep group (four muscles) (▶ Fig. 3.6).

3.2.1 Triceps Group

The long head of the triceps is the first muscle innervated by the radial nerve. Branches to this muscle arise near the axillobrachial junction. The next muscle to be innervated is the medial triceps head, followed by the lateral triceps head. This pattern of innervation is logical, considering the sequence of contact between the radial nerve and the three heads of the triceps. The main branches to the medial and lateral heads originate proximal to where the radial nerve enters the spiral groove. However, additional branches to these two muscles arise directly from the radial nerve in the spiral groove. To test the *triceps* (C6–C8), have the patient start by placing the upper arm parallel to the ground, which eliminates the effect of gravity. With the elbow half-extended, support the limb and instruct the patient to extend the elbow fully against resistance (▶ Fig. 3.7).

♦ **In about half the general population, the lateral head of the triceps is innervated prior to the medial head.**

3.2.2 Lateral Epicondyle Group

All branches to the *brachioradialis* (C5, C6) originate from the radial nerve proximal to the lateral epicondyle. To test this muscle, have the patient flex the elbow against resistance with the forearm halfway between pronation and supination (▶ Fig. 3.8). With contraction, the brachioradialis muscle becomes prominent in the lateral antecubital fossa, where it can be observed and palpated.

The two more distal muscles, the *extensor carpi radialis longus* (C6, C7) and *brevis* (C7, C8) are assessed together by having the patient extend and abduct (bend radially) the wrist against resistance while you stabilize the distal forearm (▶ Fig. 3.9). With the forearm pronated, these muscles can be seen lateral and distal to the brachioradialis. Most branches to the extensor carpi radialis longus originate from the radial nerve above the lateral epicondyle, whereas branches to the extensor carpi radialis brevis usually originate below the lateral epicondyle.

Distal to the lateral epicondyle in the proximal forearm, the posterior inter-osseous nerve innervates the *supinator* (C6, C7). Branches destined for this muscle originate from the posterior interosseous nerve prior to it passing under the arcade of Fröhse. The supinator muscle supinates the forearm. Although the biceps brachii is also a strong forearm supinator, it can be placed at a mechanical disadvantage by extending the elbow. Therefore, to isolate the supinator it should be tested with the elbow extended (▶ Fig. 3.10).

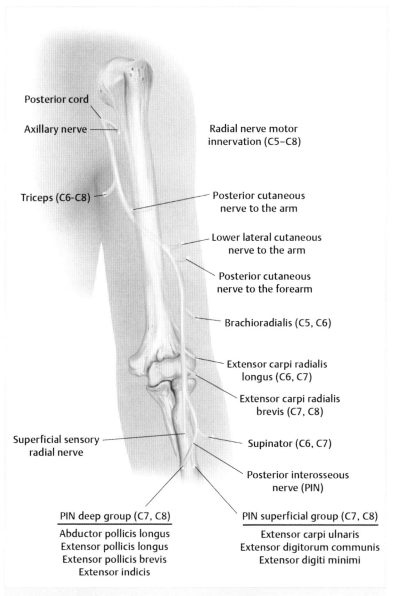

Posterior cord

Axillary nerve

Radial nerve motor
innervation (C5–C8)

Triceps (C6-C8)

Posterior cutaneous
nerve to the arm

Lower lateral cutaneous
nerve to the arm

Posterior cutaneous
nerve to the forearm

Brachioradialis (C5, C6)

Extensor carpi radialis
longus (C6, C7)

Extensor carpi radialis
brevis (C7, C8)

Superficial sensory
radial nerve

Supinator (C6, C7)

Posterior interosseous
nerve (PIN)

PIN deep group (C7, C8)
Abductor pollicis longus
Extensor pollicis longus
Extensor pollicis brevis
Extensor indicis

PIN superficial group (C7, C8)
Extensor carpi ulnaris
Extensor digitorum communis
Extensor digiti minimi

Fig. 3.6 Motor innervation of the radial nerve. The radial nerve innervates muscles that extend the forearm, hand, and fingers. It also supinates and flexes the forearm.

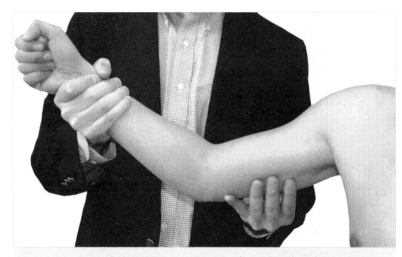

Fig. 3.7 Triceps muscle (C6–C8) assessment: Have the patient place the upper arm parallel to the ground, which eliminates the effect of gravity. Starting with the elbow half-extended, support the limb and instruct the patient to extend the elbow against resistance.

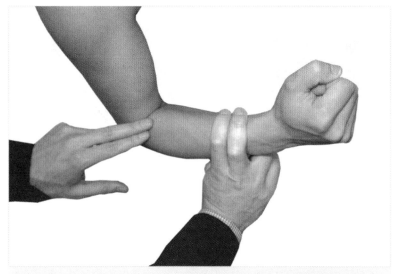

Fig. 3.8 Brachioradialis (C5, C6) assessment: The patient flexes at the elbow with the forearm halfway between pronation and supination. During contraction the brachioradialis muscle becomes prominent in the lateral antecubital fossa where it can be observed and palpated.

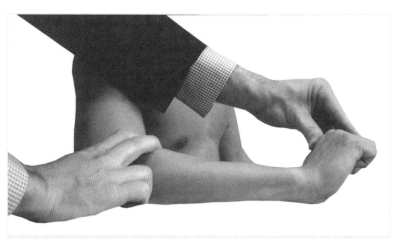

Fig. 3.9 Extensor carpi radialis longus (C6, C7) and brevis (C7, C8) assessment: These two muscles are assessed together by having the patient extend and abduct (bend radially) the wrist against resistance. With the forearm pronated, contraction of these muscles can be observed lateral and distal to the brachioradialis.

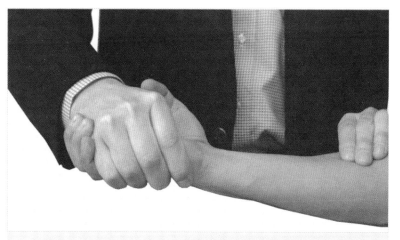

Fig. 3.10 Supinator (C6, C7) assessment: The supinator should be tested with the forearm extended, to minimize substitution by the biceps brachii. The patient maintains the forearm in supination as you attempt to pronate it.

- Because the location of the radial nerve's terminal bifurcation is variable, axons destined for the extensor carpi radialis brevis may in fact originate from either the superficial sensory radial or the posterior interosseous nerves.
- The brachialis muscle receives some innervation from the radial nerve (in addition to its main innervation from the musculocutaneous nerve). However, this innervation is usually not enough to flex the arm in the presence of a musculocutaneous nerve palsy.

3.2.3 Posterior Interosseous Nerve

Superficial Group

After passing through the supinator and entering the extensor compartment, the posterior interosseous nerve supplies the superficial group of extensor muscles, often by a common branch. This group is made up of the extensor carpi ulnaris, the extensor digitorum communis, and the extensor digiti minimi.

Test the *extensor carpi ulnaris* (C7, C8) by stabilizing the distal forearm and having the patient extend and adduct (bend in the ulnar direction) the wrist (▶ Fig. 3.11). This muscle's tendon at the wrist can be observed and palpated.

The *extensor digitorum communis* (C7, C8) extends the second to fifth digits at the metacarpal–phalangeal (knuckle) joints. To evaluate this muscle, each finger is extended at the knuckle joint, with the forearm and hand well supported in a neutral position. Apply resistance just proximal to the proximal

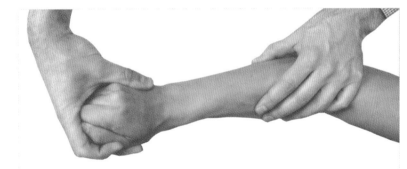

Fig. 3.11 Extensor carpi ulnaris (C7, C8) assessment: Test by stabilizing the distal forearm and having the patient extend and adduct (bend in an ulnar direction) the wrist. Its tendon can be observed and palpated at the edge of the wrist.

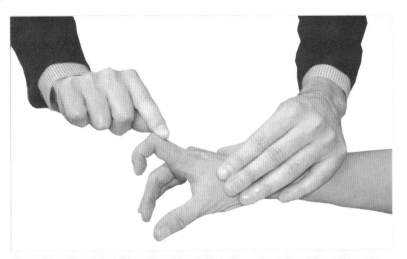

Fig. 3.12 Extensor digitorum communis (C7, C8) assessment: To evaluate this muscle, each finger is extended at the knuckle joint with the forearm and hand well supported in a neutral position. Resistance is applied just proximal to the proximal interphalangeal joint. The distal finger joints are allowed to relax in flexion.

interphalangeal joint (the distal finger joints are allowed to relax in flexion) (▶ Fig. 3.12). Another way to test finger extension at the knuckle joint is to have the patient place the hand and wrist on a flat surface and extend the fingers either together or individually. The patient should not be allowed to simultaneously flex at the wrist because this will cause the fingers to extend secondary to tenodesis (i.e., passive movement at a distal joint by changing the distance that a tendon travels by flexing or extending a more proximal joint). The second (index finger) and fifth digits (small finger) have supplementary extensors, the extensor indicis and digiti minimi, respectively. The third and fourth digits do not.

The *extensor digiti minimi* (C7, C8) acts in similar fashion as the extensor digitorum communis, yet only upon the fifth digit (▶ Fig. 3.13). This digit is normally quite weak and should be compared with the normal hand.

Deep Group

The deep group of muscles may be innervated by separate branches (more common) or via a common ("descending") branch from the posterior interosseous nerve. This group includes muscles that act upon the thumb and forefinger: abductor pollicis longus, extensor pollicis longus, extensor polli-

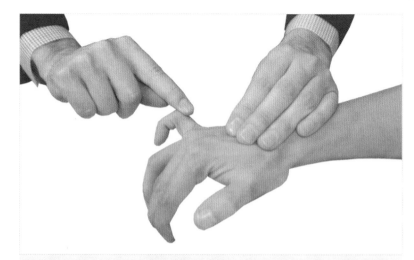

Fig. 3.13 Extensor digiti minimi (C7, C8) assessment: This muscle acts in similar fashion as the extensor digitorum communis, yet only upon the fifth digit. The fifth digit is extended at the metacarpal–phalangeal joint while its distal interphalangeal joints are relaxed in flexion.

cis brevis, and extensor indicis. These are the most distal radial-innervated muscles. Therefore, they are the last to be reinnervated following radial nerve injury.

The *abductor pollicis longus* (C7, C8) abducts the thumb in a radial direction (i.e., in the plane of the palm), unlike the median innervated abductor pollicis brevis, which primarily controls palmar abduction of the thumb (i.e., perpendicular to the plane of the palm). Therefore, one should test the abductor pollicis longus by stabilizing the hand and having the patient move an already extended thumb away from the index finger in the plane of the palm (▶ Fig. 3.14).

Thumb extension can be assessed with the hand in a fist, resting on its ulnar surface. The thumb is actively extended away from the other fingers, as if the patient was hitchhiking. The *extensor pollicis longus* (C7, C8) extends the interphalangeal joint (▶ Fig. 3.15), whereas the *extensor pollicis brevis* (C7, C8) extends the metacarpal–phalangeal joint (▶ Fig. 3.16). This can be remembered by thinking of the extensor pollicis *longus* as the "longer" of the two tendons crossing the more distal joint.

The tendons of these three thumb muscles can be seen and palpated around the anatomical "snuff box" during thumb extension. Alone, the extensor pollicis longus tendon is the distal margin of the snuff box, whereas the abductor

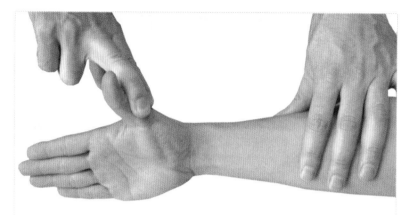

Fig. 3.14 Abductor pollicis longus (C7, C8) assessment: This muscle abducts the thumb in a radial direction (in the plane of the palm), unlike the median innervated abductor pollicis brevis, which controls palmar abduction (perpendicular to the plane of the palm). Therefore, one should test the abductor pollicis longus by stabilizing the hand and having the patient move an extended thumb away from the index finger along the plane of the palm.

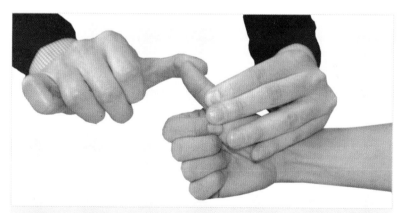

Fig. 3.15 Extensor pollicis longus (C7, C8) assessment: Thumb extension is best assessed with the hand as a fist, resting on its ulnar surface. The thumb is extended away from the other fingers, as if hitchhiking. Resistance is applied to the *distal* phalange to assess the extensor pollicis longus muscle.

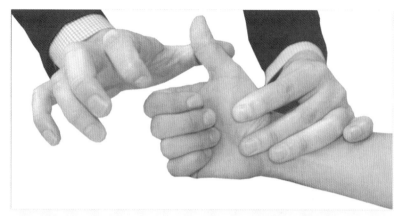

Fig. 3.16 Extensor pollicis brevis (C7, C8) assessment: Thumb extension is best assessed with the hand as a fist, resting on its ulnar surface. The thumb is extended away from the other fingers, as if hitchhiking. Resistance is applied to the *proximal* phalange to assess the extensor pollicis brevis muscle.

pollicis longus (more medial) and extensor pollicis brevis (more lateral) together form the proximal tendinous border.

The *extensor indicis* (C7, C8) acts only upon the index finger and is examined like the extensor digitorum communis (see ▶ Fig. 3.12).

♦ The posterior interosseous nerve usually ends by innervating the dorsal carpal bone joints at the wrist.
♦ Rarely, the posterior interosseous nerve can communicate with the deep motor branch of the ulnar nerve and control the first (and perhaps the first through third) dorsal interossei muscles. This anomalous extension is called the *Froment-Rauber nerve.*

3.3 Sensory Innervation

Deficits involving the radial nerve's sensory branches can help localize the level of injury. These sensory territories are depicted in ▶ Fig. 3.17.

3.3.1 Posterior Cutaneous Nerve to the Arm

The posterior cutaneous nerve to the arm is the radial nerve's first sensory branch. It originates in the axilla, passes distally with the radial nerve between the long and medial heads of the triceps, and then pierces the fascia

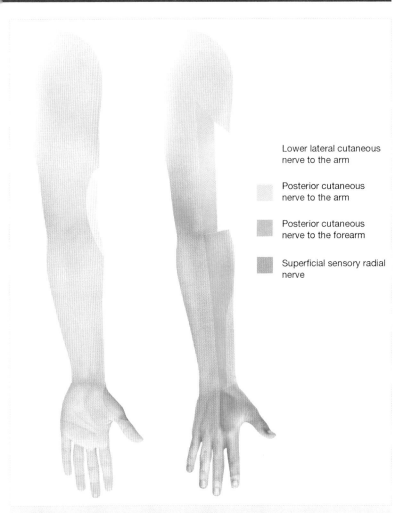

Lower lateral cutaneous
nerve to the arm

Posterior cutaneous
nerve to the arm

Posterior cutaneous
nerve to the forearm

Superficial sensory radial
nerve

Fig. 3.17 Radial nerve sensory branches. The radial nerve carries sensation from the posterior arm, lower lateral arm, posterior forearm, and dorsomedial surface of the hand. Deficits involving these sensory branches can help localize the level of radial nerve injury.

between the lateral triceps and long triceps heads to become subcutaneous. This nerve runs subcutaneously down the posterior aspect of the arm to the olecranon, a course that reflects its sensory territory. Sensory loss in the posterior arm is usually indicative of a radial nerve lesion proximal to the spiral groove.

3.3.2 Lower Lateral Cutaneous Nerve to the Arm

The lower lateral cutaneous nerve to the arm originates from the radial nerve in the spiral groove and becomes subcutaneous when it pierces the brachial fascia near the lateral intermuscular septum. This branch's sensory territory includes the lower lateral arm below the deltoid. Sensory loss here, with preserved posterior arm sensation, may indicate a radial nerve injury in the spiral groove.

3.3.3 Posterior Cutaneous Nerve to the Forearm

The posterior cutaneous nerve to the forearm branches from the radial nerve in the brachial-axillary angle, proximal to the origin of the lower lateral cutaneous nerve to the arm. The posterior cutaneous nerve to the forearm runs with the radial nerve in the spiral groove and pierces the brachial fascia with the lower lateral cutaneous nerve to the arm near the lateral intermuscular septum. Once subcutaneous, the posterior cutaneous nerve to the forearm passes posterior to the lateral epicondyle and lateral to the olecranon. Its sensory territory includes the dorsolateral aspect of the forearm.

3.3.4 Superficial Sensory Radial Nerve

As mentioned previously, the superficial sensory radial nerve runs down the forearm between the brachioradialis and extensor carpi radialis longus muscles. After becoming subcutaneous and entering the dorsum of the wrist, this nerve provides sensation to the dorsolateral half of the hand, as well as the proximal two thirds of the second, third, and lateral half of the fourth digits. The more lateral portion of the thumb is also part of this nerve's sensory territory. Opinions differ as to where the most "autonomous" zone for this nerve is located. Some include the anatomical snuff box (between the extensor pollicis longus and brevis tendons), the first dorsal web space, and the area over the distal half of the second metacarpal bone.

♦ There is much variation and overlap in sensory territories between the superficial sensory radial nerve, the dorsal ulnar cutaneous nerve, and the lateral antebrachial cutaneous nerve. Due to this overlap, isolated lesions affecting the superficial sensory radial nerve may yield a surprisingly small area of sensory loss, which may disappear over time.

For this reason, the superficial sensory radial nerve is called the *sural nerve of the arm,* and it is often harvested for graft repairs or biopsies.

3.4 Clinical Findings and Syndromes

Radial nerve deficits can be profound. Paralysis of wrist and finger extensors is debilitating because, without this movement, the hand cannot be placed in a functionally useful position. Furthermore, radial sensory deficits involving the dorsal hand, although not important for fine finger function, may be misdiagnosed and progress to refractory neuropathic pain. Triceps palsies are rare because branches to these muscles originate high in the axilla. Even when present, triceps palsies are not very disabling because gravity helps promote elbow extension. Following radial nerve injury (traumatic, idiopathic, or iatrogenic), reinnervation is frequently more robust than that seen following either median or ulnar injury. This is, in part, because the radial nerve does not innervate any distant hand intrinsic muscles. Nevertheless, radial nerve–controlled finger and thumb extension often does not return following severe, proximal radial nerve injuries. Because these movements are required for proper hand intrinsic function, their permanent paralysis becomes a common indication for tendon transfers.

3.4.1 The Arm

Complete Palsy in the Axilla

Proximal radial nerve palsies are secondary to trauma, pressure palsies, or occasionally from a posteriorly misplaced deltoid injection. Pressure palsies include crutch, Saturday night, and honeymooner's. A high radial palsy (rare) in the axilla can cause both triceps weakness and posterior arm sensory loss, two deficits that distinguish it from more common radial nerve injuries at the spiral groove. Injuries affecting the proximal radial nerve may be differentiated from posterior cord involvement by confirming normal deltoid (axillary branch off the posterior cord) and latissimus dorsi (thoracodorsal branch off the posterior cord) strength. Patients with C7 palsies can be distinguished from posterior cord or radial nerve injuries because they usually have numbness in both the volar and dorsal aspects of the third digit (middle finger), with sensory loss not extending proximal to the wrist. Additionally, C7 muscles innervated by the median nerve, including the pronator teres and flexor carpi radialis longus, would also be weak.

A complete radial palsy presents with sensory loss along the posterior arm and forearm, the lower anterolateral arm, as well as the dorsolateral hand. All extensors of the arm are weak. The triceps are weak, and the triceps reflex is

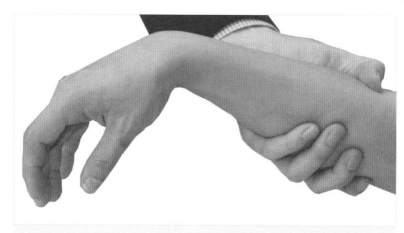

Fig. 3.18 Wrist and finger drop secondary to a radial nerve palsy. The wrist and hand appear limp with the fingers semiflexed and the first metacarpal bone (of the thumb) volar to the palm.

absent. Secondary to brachioradialis paralysis, elbow flexion may be somewhat weak compared with the normal side. There is a wrist drop from extensor carpi radialis (longus and brevis) and extensor carpi ulnaris weakness. The fingers cannot extend at the knuckle joint. Supination is partially weak, with residual supination performed by the biceps brachii. The wrist and hand appear limp, with the fingers semiflexed and the metacarpal bone of the thumb volar to the palm (▶ Fig. 3.18). Distal finger extension is possible secondary to lumbrical function.

♦ **Be aware of certain movements that may mimic true proximal finger extension. For example, when the wrist is flexed, tenodesis causes the fingers to extend. This phenomenon may be exaggerated when sclerosis is present from chronic extensor paralysis. Furthermore, with the fingers partially flexed, the hand intrinsics may partially extend the knuckle joints. To remove these effects, examine metacarpal joint extension with the wrist held in extension or stabilized on a flat surface.**

Radial Nerve Damage in the Spiral Groove

The spiral groove is the most common location for traumatic radial nerve palsy. The radial nerve can be directly contused against the humerus, or damaged by a fracture of the midhumeral shaft. It is estimated that approximately 15% of

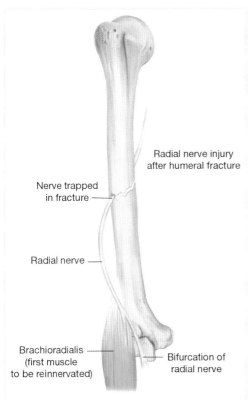

Fig. 3.19 Radial nerve injury following a humeral fracture. With a humeral fracture, the radial nerve remains tethered to the lateral intermuscular septum; this immobility can pin it between the two ends of fractured bone.

Radial nerve injury after humeral fracture

Nerve trapped in fracture

Radial nerve

Brachioradialis (first muscle to be reinnervated)

Bifurcation of radial nerve

midhumeral fractures affect the radial nerve. With a humeral fracture, the radial nerve remains tethered where it pierces the lateral intermuscular septum, and due to this immobility, it may become caught between the fractured ends of bone (► Fig. 3.19). A distally misplaced deltoid injection may also damage the radial nerve in this region.

Radial nerve lesions at the spiral groove cause weakness of all radial-innervated muscles distal to the elbow, including the brachioradialis. The triceps are usually spared, as is the triceps reflex. Loss of sensation along the lower lateral arm and posterior forearm usually occurs, whereas the posterior cutaneous nerve to the arm is spared because it does not run in the spiral groove. The brachioradialis is the most proximal muscle to be reinnervated following radial nerve injury at the spiral groove, a process that usually takes 3 to 4 months.

♦ In some patients, damage to the radial nerve at the spiral groove may cause mild triceps weakness. This is because supplementary branches to the lateral and medial heads from the radial nerve originate in the spiral groove, where they may be injured.

3.4.2 The Antecubital Fossa

Radial Tunnel Syndrome

The existence of radial tunnel syndrome remains controversial. This is because, by definition, this syndrome has no objective motor or sensory deficits on examination or electrodiagnostic studies. If these are present, especially finger extension weakness, one must consider other diagnoses, specifically posterior interosseous nerve compression at the supinator. Anatomically, the radial tunnel is the submuscular path where the radial nerve travels between the lateral intermuscular septum and the supinator. Between these two points, the brachioradialis, extensor carpi radialis longus, and extensor carpi radialis brevis muscles sequentially cover the radial nerve. The extensor carpi radialis brevis actually envelops the nerve by passing both deep and superficial to it. Some experts propose that irritation of the radial nerve in the radial tunnel can be secondary to an anomalous tendinous ridge on the extensor carpi radialis brevis muscle. Other compression points may include fibrous bands on the anterior margin of the elbow joint and/or radial head, or alternatively, from a fan of small arterial branches off the recurrent radial artery.

Radial tunnel syndrome and tennis elbow (i.e., lateral epicondylitis) have very similar presentations. Diagnostic criteria for radial tunnel syndrome include: (1) lack of response to conservative treatment of tennis elbow, (2) pain worsening at the radial tunnel (not the lateral epicondyle) during resisted third digit extension when the elbow is fully extended and the forearm supinated, and (3) tenderness in the radial tunnel at rest. The third digit is believed to instigate pain because the extensor carpi radialis brevis inserts on the third metacarpal bone (the extensor carpi radialis longus inserts on the second). Forced supination may also cause pain if the radial tunnel is simultaneously palpated.

♦ In contrast, tennis elbow is secondary to forced, repetitive pronation and wrist extension causing inflammation where the extensor muscles attach to the lateral epicondyle. Relief of symptoms with a cortisone injection at the lateral epicondyle is often diagnostic. Patients with tennis elbow have pain at the lateral epicondyle, not the radial tunnel, and classically have worsened pain when the hand is passively pronated and flexed (placing the tendinous insertions on stretch). Tennis elbow pain is often sharp and localized, whereas for radial tunnel syndrome, there is a dull ache deep in the muscles.

Supinator Syndrome

Supinator syndrome is a posterior interosseous nerve palsy secondary to compression where this nerve enters the supinator. The posterior interosseous nerve passes between the superficial and deep heads of this muscle, analogous to placing your index finger into the front pocket of a pair of jeans. The anterior margin of this "pocket" is termed the arcade of Fröhse, and in 30% of the general population it is fibrous and thought to cause nerve compression (▶ Fig. 3.20). Some patients with this syndrome have a history of mild trauma

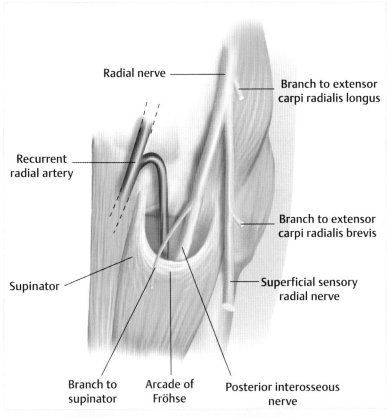

Fig. 3.20 Supinator syndrome. The posterior interosseous nerve may be compressed where it enters the supinator. It passes between the superficial and deep heads of this muscle, analogous to placing your index finger into the front pocket of a pair of jeans. The anterior margin of this "pocket" is called the *arcade of Fröhse*, which may be fibrous and can cause compression.

to the forearm, or, alternatively, they report repetitive supination movements prior to onset.

Patients with supinator syndrome often have pain localized to the supinator muscle, which worsens after a few minutes of forced supination. By history, they have either sudden or progressive finger extension weakness. Denervation of the supinator is classically spared in supinator syndrome because most branches to this muscle occur prior to the nerve passing under the arcade of Fröhse. Sensation is normal in the territory of the superficial sensory radial nerve, and the brachioradialis muscle has normal strength. Some believe that many patients diagnosed with this syndrome instead have a focal case of inflammatory neuritis (i.e., Parsonage-Turner syndrome).

♦ **The healing of a proximal forearm or elbow fracture in misalignment, or with excessive pannus, may put the posterior interosseous nerve, which is relatively fixed at its entrance into the supinator muscle, under tension. The resultant palsy, termed tardive radial palsy, usually presents months to years later. It classically occurs after a Monteggia fracture: a proximal ulnar fracture with concurrent posterior disloca-tion of the radius. Radiographs are diagnostic.**

♦ **Patients with rheumatoid arthritis are predisposed to finger exten-sion weakness. They can have synovial thickening at the elbow that compresses the radial nerve directly or indirectly by elevating the supinator, which places the posterior interosseous nerve on stretch. Rheumatoid arthritis patients can also rupture extensor tendons, which can mimic nerve palsy.**

3.4.3 The Forearm

Posterior Interosseous Nerve Palsy

Posterior interosseous nerve palsy can be from trauma, diabetic mono-neuropathy, compression at the supinator muscle (supinator syndrome), or a space-occupying mass, or as a manifestation of Parsonage-Turner syn-drome. The most common soft tissue mass compressing the posterior interosseous nerve is a lipoma, followed by nerve sheath tumors, ganglion cysts, and hypertrophic synovium (rheumatoid arthritis). Considering it carries no cutaneous sensory fibers, sensation remains normal. However, patients may complain of a dull ache in the proximal forearm extensor muscles near the radial head.

Posterior interosseous nerve palsy has two components: wrist extension weakness in an ulnar direction (radial wrist extension remains normal, medi-ated by the extensor carpi radialis longus and brevis), and finger extension weakness at the metacarpal–phalangeal joints. Of note, patients do *not* have a wrist drop because the two extensor carpi radialis muscles are unaffected.

Upon wrist extension, however, the hand may deviate in a radial direction because the extensor carpi ulnaris is weak. Isolated posterior interosseous nerve palsy is confirmed by documenting normal brachioradialis and superficial sensory radial nerve function. Patients with partial posterior interosseous nerve lesions can have variable weakness in each finger. When weakness occurs in only the fourth and fifth digits, a pseudo–ulnar claw hand can develop. However, there is no hyperextension at the knuckle joints, which differentiates it from a true claw hand.

♦ Supinator and extensor carpi radialis brevis weakness may occur from a posterior interosseous nerve palsy if the injury is proximal to the arcade of Fröhse.

3.4.4 Sensory Radial Nerve Palsy (Wartenberg Syndrome)

Isolated damage to the superficial sensory radial nerve can occur from trauma, tight handcuffs or watches, venipuncture, surgery for de Quervain teno-

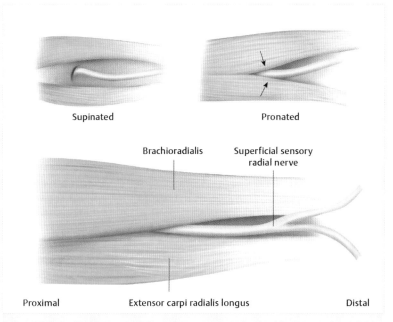

Fig. 3.21 Superficial sensory radial nerve entrapment in the distal forearm. With repetitive pronation, the brachioradialis tendon normally closes the space between these two tendons in a scissor-like fashion, potentially irritating the nerve where it emerges from the fascia.

synovitis, and occasionally from scissor-like pinching between the brachioradialis and extensor carpi radialis longus tendons. *Wartenberg syndrome* and *cheiralgia paresthetica* are synonymous with *superficial sensory radial nerve palsy*. It is defined by numbness, hyperesthesia, and burning pain on the dorsolateral aspect of the hand. With misdiagnosis and lack of treatment, this pain may become permanent and therefore difficult to treat. The superficial sensory radial nerve pierces the antebrachial fascia approximately two thirds down the forearm at the lateral (radial) border, between the tendons of the brachioradialis and extensor carpi radialis longus (▶ Fig. 3.21). During pronation, the brachioradialis tendon closes the space between these two tendons in a scissor-like fashion, potentially irritating the nerve where it pierces the fascia. In these patients, pain and numbness can be exacerbated by forced pronation and ulnar wrist deviation, which scissors the tendons together and stretches the nerve, respectively. A Tinel sign can often be elicited. This diagnosis may be confirmed with electrodiagnostic testing.

♦ De Quervain tenosynovitis, or stenosing tenosynovitis of the first thumb's extensor tendon, may be confused with superficial sensory radial nerve palsy because they both can cause pain near the wrist. The *Finkelstein sign* for de Quervain tenosynovitis occurs if passively bending the hand (as a fist) in an ulnar direction causes pain in the lateral wrist area. A superficial sensory radial nerve palsy may also have a positive Finkelstein sign. Sensory loss, however, differentiates them: it is usually absent in stenosing tenosynovitis.

4 Brachial Plexus Anatomy

4.1 Proximal Brachial Plexus

4.1.1 Nerves and Trunks

The brachial plexus is composed of axons from five spinal nerves: C5, C6, C7, C8, and T1. Starting in the spinal canal, multiple ventral (motor) and dorsal (sensory) rootlets exit the spinal cord and coalesce into motor and sensory roots before entering the intervertebral foramina. In the proximal intervertebral foramen, the sensory root enters its spinal ganglion. At the midportion of the intervertebral foramen, the motor and sensory roots merge to form a single spinal nerve. This merger is short-lived, however, because the spinal nerve almost immediately splits into ventral and dorsal rami upon exiting the foramen. The dorsal rami exit posteriorly to innervate the paraspinal muscles and skin; the ventral rami form the brachial plexus.

As a spinal nerve passes through the intervertebral foramen, its enveloping dura gradually turns into epineurium. The primary site of adherence, or stabilization, of spinal nerves is just outside the foramen, where the inferior aspect of the nerve is attached to a depression in the transverse process. This is the only bony attachment of the brachial plexus, and it serves to protect the weak intradural rootlets from traction injury, thereby preventing their avulsion from the spinal cord. This attachment is well developed for C5, C6, and C7, but it is weak or absent for C8 and T1, making these latter two nerves more susceptible to avulsion injury.

Immediately after the ventral rami form, prior to entering the brachial plexus, they communicate with the sympathetic ganglia. This connection with the sympathetic nervous system includes both gray and white rami. More proximally, the gray ramus carries postsynaptic fibers from the sympathetic ganglia to the spinal nerve; they are destined for sweat glands and vasoconstrictors. The slightly more distal white ramus carries preganglionic information from the spinal cord to the sympathetic ganglia.

Of importance, the sympathetic fibers destined for the face via the trigeminal nerve originate from the upper thoracic spinal cord, travel through the T1 and T2 spinal nerves, and pass via the white rami into the paravertebral ganglia. These sympathetic axons travel cranially, ultimately terminating in the superior cervical ganglion. Postsynaptic sympathetic axons exit this ganglion and enter the head upon the internal carotid artery, only to be subsequently transferred to the trigeminal nerve in the cavernous sinus. Following the branches of the trigeminal nerve, these axons mediate facial sweating, pupillary dilatation, and contraction of both the tarsal muscles and the Müller muscle. Therefore, damage to the T1 or T2 spinal nerve can cause *Horner syndrome:* anhidrosis (lack of sweating), miosis (lack of pupillary dilatation), ptosis (tarsal muscle weakness), and enophthalmos (palsy of the Müller muscle). The presence of Horner syndrome is a sign of very proximal injury to the brachial plexus or the spinal nerves or both.

The two upper spinal nerves, C5 and C6, merge to become the upper trunk. The lower two spinal nerves, C8 and T1, travel a bit cranially over the first rib to form the lower trunk. This leaves C7 alone to create the middle trunk. These three trunks (upper, middle, and lower), once formed, travel distally toward the clavicle (▶ Fig. 4.1). Excluding variations, the only branches from the proximal brachial plexus originate from the C5, C6, and C7 spinal nerves, as well as the upper trunk; whereas the middle and lower trunks, as well as the C8 and T1 spinal nerves, usually do not have any branches of clinical significance.

From the spine to the clavicle, the spinal nerves and trunks run sandwiched between the anterior and middle scalene muscles (the scalenes). The only components of the supraclavicular brachial plexus not completely covered by these two muscles are C5, C6, and a proximal portion of the upper trunk. The point where C5 and C6 merge to create the upper trunk is called the *Erb's point.* C8 and T1 start below the scalenes, but they rise cranially to be flanked by them.

♦ Prior to entering the brachial plexus, the spinal nerves are commonly referred to as roots. Although this nomenclature is not correct, it is commonly used.

♦ Occasionally, either C4 or T2 may contribute to the brachial plexus. When there is C4 contribution and a small T1 input, the brachial plexus is considered *prefixed.* However, when there is minor C5 spinal nerve input with a definite T2 contribution, the plexus is considered *postfixed.*

4.1.2 Spinal Nerve Branches

Prior to entering the upper trunk, three nerves receive input from the C5 nerve root: the phrenic nerve to the diaphragm, the long thoracic nerve to the serratus anterior, and the dorsal scapular nerve to the rhomboid muscles. C6 and C7 also provide fibers to the long thoracic nerve (▶ Fig. 4.2). As mentioned, no important branches usually arise from the C8 and T1 spinal nerves.

Phrenic Nerve

The C5 spinal nerve provides input to the phrenic nerve. The phrenic nerve is made up of motor axons from the C3, C4, and C5 spinal nerves; hence the phrase "C3, 4, and 5 keeps a person alive." After being formed, the phrenic nerve runs distally on the superficial aspect of the anterior scalene muscle, somewhat lateral to medial (it is the only nerve that runs lateral to medial in the posterior triangle). With the anterior scalene, the phrenic nerve passes between the subclavian artery (located posterior) and the subclavian vein

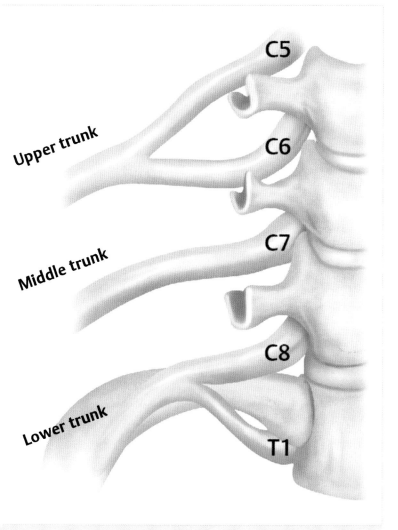

Fig. 4.1 Proximal brachial plexus: spinal nerves to trunks without branches. The two upper spinal nerves, C5 and C6, merge to become the upper trunk, whereas the lower two spinal nerves, C8 and T1, travel cranially over the first rib to form the lower trunk. This leaves only C7 to create the middle trunk.

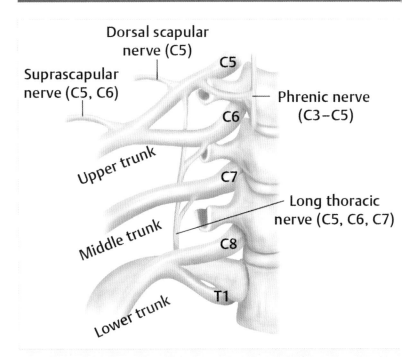

Fig. 4.2 Proximal brachial plexus: spinal nerves to trunks with branches. Three branches receive a contribution from the C5 nerve: the phrenic, long thoracic, and dorsal scapular. C6 and C7 also contribute to the long thoracic nerve. One important branch originates from the upper trunk: the suprascapular nerve.

(located anterior) when entering the thorax. Each phrenic nerve innervates one *hemidiaphragm.* Depending on the amount of C5 input within the phrenic nerve, a proximal C5 nerve root injury may cause an ipsilaterally elevated and paralyzed diaphragm. This may be diagnosed by comparing the percussion of both lungs during inspiration. A radiograph or ultrasound will also confirm this type of paralysis.

Phrenic nerve damage may occur during open-heart surgery secondary to the use of ice slush to cool the heart. When this occurs, it is thought to be a cause of respirator dependence, especially when bilateral palsies are present.

Long Thoracic Nerve

Another branch from the proximal brachial plexus prior to trunk formation is the long thoracic nerve, having intraforaminal contributions from C5, C6 and C7. The long thoracic nerve forms dorsal to the spinal nerves, travels behind the proximal brachial plexus caudally between the anterior and middle scalenes over the posterolateral portion of the first rib, eventually innervating the *serratus anterior* muscle. The serratus anterior pulls the scapula away from midline and forward around the thorax (scapular abduction). It also rotates the scapula upward. Most importantly, however, this muscle fixes and stabilizes the scapula so that muscles originating from it can function properly.

Injury to the long thoracic nerve causes scapular winging. At rest with serratus anterior weakness, there may be prominence of the scapula's inferomedial edge, with medial displacement and downward rotation. Winging is classically worsened when the patient pushes forward against resistance, with the elbow fully extended and the shoulder girdle protracted forward (anterior) (▶ Fig. 4.3). This latter finding is the hallmark of a long thoracic palsy.

To test the serratus anterior, instruct the patient to reach forward to a point on the wall, and then apply resistance at the hand or wrist while stabilizing the thorax with the other hand. A common mistake is to not have the patient displace the shoulder girdle forward enough, because without doing so scapular winging from trapezius or rhomboid weakness may be misdiagnosed as a long thoracic palsy. Of note, weakness of any of these three muscles can cause scapular winging when the arm is pushed against resistance across the chest with the arm bent.

- **Sometimes there is no C7 spinal nerve input to the long thoracic nerve.**
- **Weakness itself of the serratus anterior often causes a dull ache in the shoulder region. However, if the pain is relatively sudden and severe, one should consider acute brachial neuritis.**

Dorsal Scapular Nerve

The dorsal scapular nerve originates from the C5 spinal nerve, usually without input from other spinal nerves. It innervates both the major and the minor *rhomboid muscles* (the rhomboids). The rhomboids connect the medial edge of the scapula to the spinal column. When contracted, the rhomboids pull the scapula toward midline (scapular adduction) and elevate its medial border cranially (i.e., downward scapular rotation)—opposing the serratus anterior. The dorsal scapular nerve passes dorsal to the brachial plexus, eventually perforating the middle scalene. It then travels along the undersurface of the levator scapulae down to the rhomboids. With chronic denervation of the rhomboids, interscapular wasting is evident. With rhomboid weakness, there may be mild scapular winging at rest, especially at the inferomedial edge. The scapula may also be laterally displaced. To test the rhomboids, have the patient place the palm on the lower back facing outward. Instruct the patient to push

Brachial Plexus Anatomy

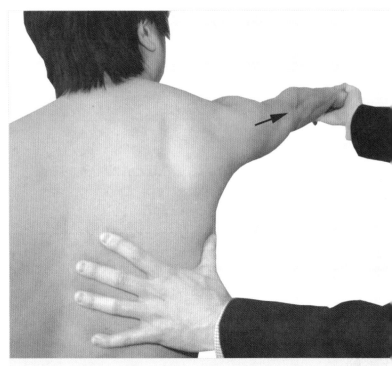

Fig. 4.3 Serratus anterior (C5, C6, C7) assessment: Instruct the patient to reach forward to a point on the wall, and then apply resistance at the wrist while stabilizing the thorax with your other hand. A common mistake is to not have the patient displace the shoulder girdle forward enough (i.e., not enough shoulder protraction), because, without doing so, scapular winging from trapezius or rhomboid weakness may be misdiagnosed as a long thoracic palsy.

the palm away from the lower back as you apply resistance to the hand as well as to the arm (apply resistance in an anterolateral direction around the thorax) (▶ Fig. 4.4). Observe and palpate the rhomboids during this maneuver. Concurrent damage to the proximal brachial plexus is often present; therefore, the forearm may need to be supported. An alternate method to examine the rhomboids is to have the patient bring the shoulders and scapulae together posteriorly. In this position, the contracted rhomboids can be palpated between the medial aspects of the scapulae.

♦ **The dorsal scapular nerve can provide partial innervation to the levator scapula as it passes underneath this muscle.**

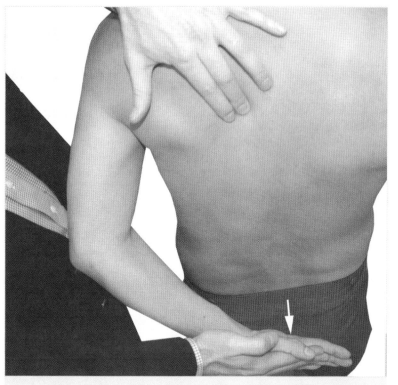

Fig. 4.4 Major and minor rhomboids (C5) assessment: Have the patient place the palm facing outward on the lower back. Instruct the patient to push the palm away from the lower back as you apply resistance to the hand as well as to the arm (the arm is pushed anterior and lateral around the thorax). Instruct the patient to lead with the hand, not the elbow.

4.1.3 Truncal Branches

There is only one branch of significance from the brachial plexus trunks: the suprascapular nerve. This nerve originates from the distal, superior aspect of the upper trunk, just above the clavicle. In summary, all the proximal brachial plexus branches come from the C5, C6, and C7 spinal nerves, or the upper trunk, with C5 input being present in all of them (see ▶ Fig. 4.2).

Suprascapular Nerve

The *suprascapular nerve* (C5, C6) descends posteriorly and distally along the superior portion of the upper trunk. It subsequently passes between the

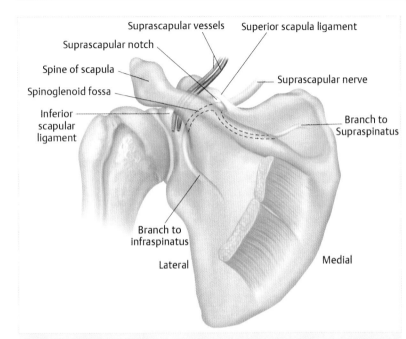

Fig. 4.5 Suprascapular anatomy. The suprascapular nerve passes under the superior scapular ligament; the artery and vein pass over this ligament. This neurovascular bundle then passes around the lateral edge of the scapular spine through the spinoglenoid fossa. Here both the vessels and nerve pass under the inferior scapular ligament.

inferior belly of the omohyoid and the trapezius muscle toward the suprascapular notch. The suprascapular nerve's convergence with the omohyoid muscle at the scapula confirms its identity during surgical exposure. The suprascapular artery and vein traverse the brachial plexus just superior and deep to the clavicle, joining the suprascapular nerve as it approaches the suprascapular notch. The suprascapular nerve passes through the notch and under the superior scapular ligament; the artery and vein pass over this ligament (▶ Fig. 4.5). The nerve and vessels once again join as they pass around the lateral edge of the scapular spine through the spinoglenoid fossa. Here, all components of the neurovascular bundle pass under the inferior scapular ligament. The suprascapular nerve innervates the *suprascapular* and *infraspinatus* muscles. The suprascapular attaches to the superior aspect of the humeral head and mediates the initial 20 to 30 degrees of arm abduction. The infraspinatus attaches to the posterior aspect of the humeral head and is the primary external rotator of the arm. Test the suprascapular muscle by having the patient abduct a straight arm, starting at the patient's side, against resistance (▶ Fig. 4.6). To test the infraspinatus muscle, start with the patient flexing the elbow to 90 degrees. Then stabilize the elbow against the patient's side and ask the patient to rotate the arm externally against resistance, like a tennis swing (▶ Fig. 4.7). Contraction of the supraspinatus and infraspinatus muscles can be observed and palpated during testing. With chronic denervation, atrophy above (supraspinatus) or below (infraspinatus) the scapular spine is readily appreciated.

Acute suprascapular palsies are usually secondary to trauma (abrupt shoulder distraction or scapular fractures); therefore, for gradual-onset palsy one should consider a ganglion cyst or idiopathic entrapment at the suprascapular notch. If there is a great deal of shoulder pain that improves as muscle weakness appears, then acute brachial neuritis is likely. For entrapment cases, narrowing or callus involving the suprascapular notch may be seen on properly directed radiographs.

♦ **The small, often forgotten, subclavius nerve to the subclavius muscle also originates from the upper trunk. This muscle, however, cannot be tested clinically or electrophysiologically.**

4.2 Distal Brachial Plexus

4.2.1 Major Branches from the Cords

The distal portion of the brachial plexus is composed of cords, which are named according to their relationship to the axillary artery deep to the pectoralis minor muscle (lateral, medial, posterior) (▶ Fig. 4.8). The cords are intimately associated with the axillary artery and vein in this region. As the brachial plexus cords pass further distal to the pectoralis minor, their anatomical relationship to this artery changes—they are no longer lateral, medial, and posterior.

The major, terminal branches of the brachial plexus have been discussed in Chapters 1, 2, and 3 (i.e., median, ulnar, and radial nerves). The median nerve is not a continuation of any cord per se, but is created from a lateral contribution from the lateral cord (mostly sensory), as well as a medial contribution from the medial cord (mostly motor to hand intrinsics). Both of these contributions pass superficial to the axillary artery and form the median nerve on its anterior surface. After giving these contributions, the remaining portion of the medial cord continues into the arm as the ulnar nerve; the remaining portion of the lateral cord continues as the musculocutaneous nerve. This anatomical arrangement resembles an M over the axillary, then brachial artery, with the center leg being the median nerve, the lateral leg the musculocutaneous nerve, and the medial leg the ulnar nerve. The posterior cord runs deep to the axillary artery, with the axillary nerve branching prior to it continuing as the radial nerve. The musculocutaneous and axillary nerves will be discussed next.

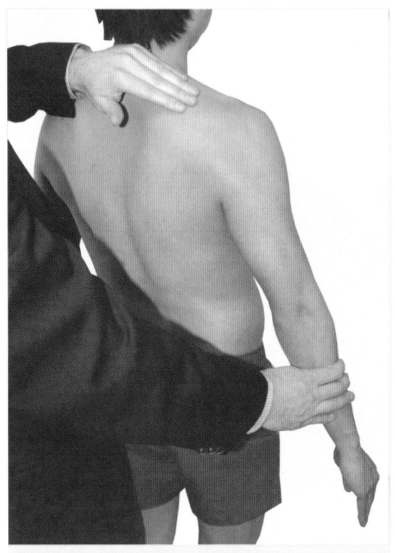

Fig. 4.6 Supraspinatus (C5, C6) assessment: Test the supraspinatus muscle by having the patient abduct a straight arm from the side against resistance.

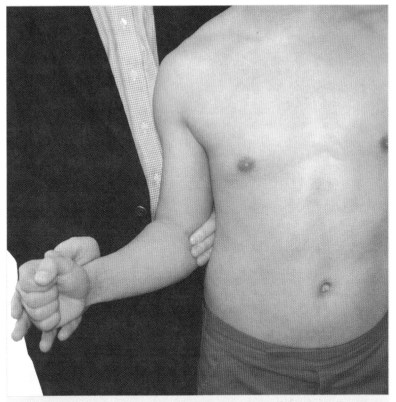

Fig. 4.7 Infraspinatus (C5, C6) assessment: Start with the patient flexing the elbow to 90 degrees. Then stabilize the elbow against the patient's side and ask the patient to rotate the arm externally against resistance, like a tennis swing (the teres minor also externally rotates the arm).

4.2.2 The Musculocutaneous Nerve

The *musculocutaneous nerve* (C5, C6) is the distal continuation of the lateral cord containing axons from the upper trunk (▶ Fig. 4.9). In the axilla, the musculocutaneous nerve travels distal and somewhat lateral to pierce the *coracobrachialis* muscle, which it innervates. The coracobrachialis muscle assists the anterior deltoid with shoulder flexion (lifting the arm forward in front of the body). It also stabilizes the humerus during elbow flexion. The coracobrachialis cannot be isolated or readily palpated. Therefore, it is not examined clinically. After passing through and then deep to the coracobrachialis, the

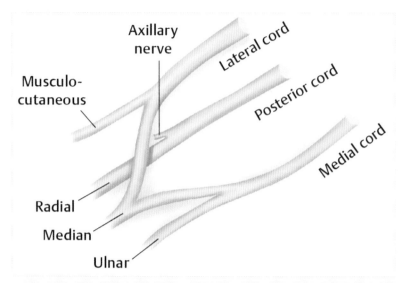

Fig. 4.8 Distal brachial plexus cords and terminal branches. The distal portion of the brachial plexus is composed of cords, which are named according to their relationship to the axillary artery deep to the pectoralis minor (lateral, medial, posterior).

musculocutaneous nerve continues on the superficial surface of the *brachialis* muscle deep to the *biceps brachii.* These two muscles are innervated via multiple branches off the musculocutaneous nerve. Distally, the musculocutaneous nerve enters the antecubital fossa, where it pierces the superficial fascia just lateral to the biceps tendon, entering the subcutaneous space as the *lateral antebrachial cutaneous nerve.* The territory of this sensory nerve includes, as the name implies, the lateral half of the forearm (▶ Fig. 4.10). The lateral antebrachial cutaneous nerve has anterior and posterior divisions.

The biceps brachii, with the assistance of the brachialis and brachioradialis, flexes the elbow. The biceps brachii is also a strong supinator of the forearm when the elbow is flexed. To test the biceps brachii and brachialis, have the patient flex a fully supinated forearm against resistance (▶ Fig. 4.11). Contribution from the brachioradialis is minimized by testing with the forearm in full supination.

Isolated musculocutaneous palsies are rare but can occur following trauma or shoulder dislocation. These patients present with numbness in their anterolateral forearm, along with elbow flexion weakness. These findings need to be clinically differentiated from a biceps tendon rupture, as well as from a C6 radiculopathy. Following tendon rupture, the biceps still contracts and can be felt rolling up the arm. A C6 radiculopathy is identified not only

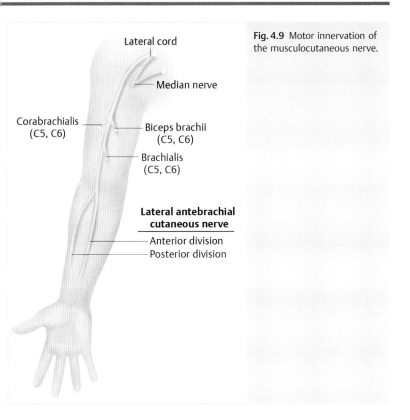

Fig. 4.9 Motor innervation of the musculocutaneous nerve.

Lateral cord

Median nerve

Corabrachialis
(C5, C6)

Biceps brachii
(C5, C6)

Brachialis
(C5, C6)

Lateral antebrachial cutaneous nerve

Anterior division
Posterior division

because of the radicular pain but also because of possible weakness in other, nonmusculocutaneous innervated, C6 muscles, including the brachioradialis and latissimus dorsi. Furthermore, C6 radiculopathies usually cause numbness confined to the thumb and index finger, whereas the sensory coverage of the lateral antebrachial cutaneous nerve stops at the wrist. Focal damage to the lateral antebrachial cutaneous nerve can be from venipuncture in the antecubital fossa.

4.2.3 The Axillary Nerve

The *axillary nerve* (C5, C6) arises from the posterior cord deep to the axillary artery. A branch off the axillary artery, the posterior humeral circumflex artery, joins the axillary nerve, passing inferior and medial to it. This neurovascular bundle travels briefly upon the subscapularis muscle toward the surgical neck of the humerus. It then passes through the *quadrangular, or quadrilateral, space,*

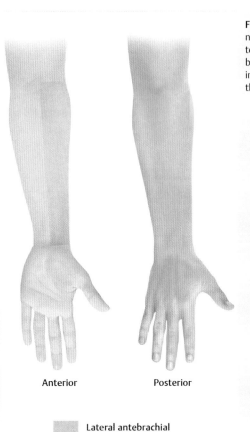

Fig. 4.10 Musculocutaneous nerve sensory territory. The territory of the lateral antebrachial cutaneous nerve includes, as the name implies, the lateral half of the forearm.

Anterior   Posterior

Lateral antebrachial cutaneous nerve

which is bordered superiorly by the teres minor, inferiorly by the teres major, laterally by the neck of the humerus, and medially by the long head of the triceps (▶ Fig. 4.12). The axillary nerve is relatively fixed at the quadrangular space, and, analogous to the suprascapular nerve in the suprascapular notch, is vulnerable to stretch injury when blunt or traction forces are applied to the brachial plexus or shoulder. Immediately after passing through the quadrangular space, the axillary nerve divides into anterior and posterior divisions. The anterior division curves anterior and somewhat superior under the *deltoid muscle,* which it innervates. The posterior division gives an immediate branch to the *teres minor* after passing through the quadrangular space (▶ Fig. 4.13). The posterior division then pierces the brachial fascia distal and posterior to the deltoid's insertion into the humerus

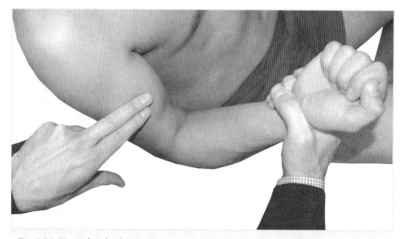

Fig. 4.11 Biceps brachii (C5, C6) assessment: To test the biceps brachii and brachialis, have the patient flex a fully supinated forearm against resistance. By testing the forearm in full supination, contribution from the brachioradialis (radial nerve) is minimized.

to become cutaneous. This cutaneous portion of the axillary nerve carries sensation from the upper lateral arm (► Fig. 4.14); it is called the *upper lateral brachial cutaneous nerve.* The axillary nerve also carries sensory fibers from the shoulder joint.

The teres minor assists the infraspinatus in externally rotating the arm. It also weakly assists the teres major in adducting a straight arm. It is not possible to test the teres minor in complete isolation, but one may observe and palpate its contraction if the patient is thin. The deltoid is the prime abductor of the arm, especially between 30 and 90 degrees. The initial 30 degrees of abduction is primarily controlled by the supraspinatus, whereas abduction above 90 degrees has an important trapezial component, a muscle that rotates the shoulder girdle upward. Test the deltoid by having the patient abduct the arm against resistance (► Fig. 4.15). The deltoid has three separate heads: the anterior, lateral, and posterior. Abducting the arm to the side and slightly in front of the body tests the anterior and lateral heads of the deltoid. To assess the posterior head, have the patient place a straightened arm almost 90 degrees abducted, and then ask the patient to move the arm posterior and superior against resistance (► Fig. 4.16). The absence of posterior deltoid contraction can help confirm an axillary palsy, especially in those patients with a powerful supraspinatus muscle that alone can abduct the arm to 90 degrees. Arm flexion at the shoulder (in front of the body) is mediated by the anterior deltoid. Although the initial 60 degrees of arm flexion is mostly

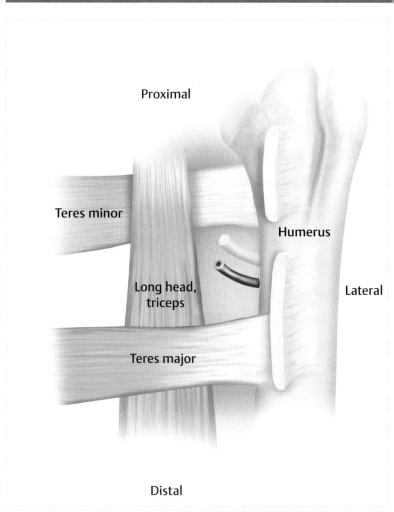

Fig. 4.12 Borders of the quadrangular space, ventral perspective. The axillary nerve passes through the quadrangular space, which is bordered superiorly by the teres minor, inferiorly by the teres major, laterally by the neck of the humerus, and medially by the long head of the triceps.

anterior deltoid, the serratus anterior assists the deltoid during flexion above 60 degrees.

The axillary nerve is usually injured in isolation by shoulder trauma, including shoulder dislocations or humeral fractures. For patients with suspected

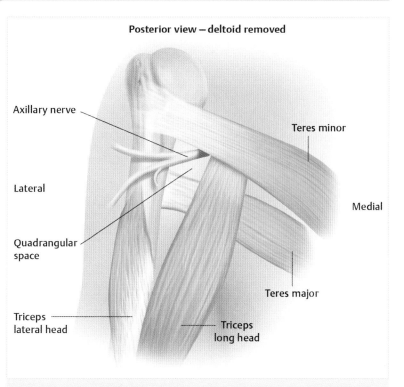

Posterior view – deltoid removed

Axillary nerve

Teres minor

Lateral

Medial

Quadrangular space

Teres major

Triceps lateral head

Triceps long head

Fig. 4.13 Axillary nerve anatomy, posterior view with deltoid removed. Immediately after passing through the quadrangular space, the axillary nerve divides into anterior and posterior divisions. The anterior division curves anterior and somewhat superior under the deltoid muscle, which it innervates. The posterior division gives an immediate branch to the teres minor after passing through the quadrangular space, and then becomes subcutaneous by piercing the brachial fascia.

axillary neuropathy following shoulder trauma, one should always exclude partial damage to the posterior division of the brachial plexus as an alternate diagnosis. By examining the latissimus dorsi (the thoracodorsal nerve), as well as all the muscles innervated by the radial nerve, posterior cord involvement can be excluded. The axillary nerve may be compressed at the quadrangular space, which is known as the *quadrangular space syndrome.* The etiology of this entrapment is uncertain.

♦ Even with complete deltoid paralysis, patients may use other upper-extremity muscles to abduct the arm, thereby mimicking deltoid function. As mentioned, a well-developed supraspinatus can

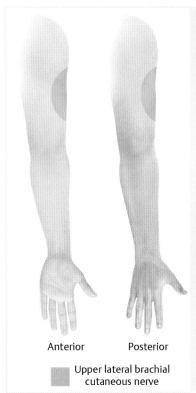

Fig. 4.14 Axillary nerve sensory territory. The posterior division of the axillary nerve ends by piercing the brachial fascia distal and posterior to the deltoid's insertion into the humerus. This cutaneous extension of the axillary nerve carries sensation from the upper lateral arm and is called the *upper lateral brachial cutaneous nerve*.

Anterior Posterior

Upper lateral brachial cutaneous nerve

achieve more than 30 degrees of arm abduction. The external rotators of the arm may also weakly abduct the arm. In addition, both the coracobrachialis and the long head of the triceps, which connect the scapula to the humerus and olecranon, respectively, can substitute for deltoid function by lifting the arm. Therefore, palpating the deltoid during muscle testing is important.

4.3 Distal Brachial Plexus

4.3.1 Minor Branches from the Cords

Aside from the major terminal branches described in the previous section (e.g., musculocutaneous and axillary nerves), each cord has other smaller, "minor" branches (▶ Fig. 4.17). Damage to any of these branches helps localize a lesion to the cord level.

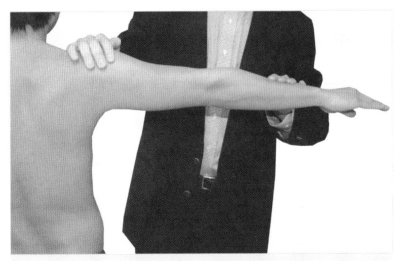

Fig. 4.15 Deltoid (C5, C6) assessment: Test the deltoid by having the patient abduct the arm against resistance. The deltoid has three separate heads: anterior, lateral, and posterior. Abducting the arm to the side, and slightly in front of the body, tests the anterior and lateral heads of the deltoid. The deltoid controls abduction between 30 and 90 degrees.

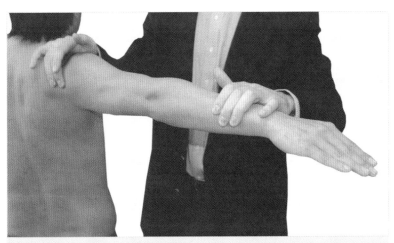

Fig. 4.16 Posterior deltoid (C5, C6) assessment: To assess the posterior deltoid, have the patient place a straightened arm almost 90 degrees abducted, and then ask the patient to move the arm posteriorly and superiorly against resistance. Contraction of the posterior head can be observed and palpated.

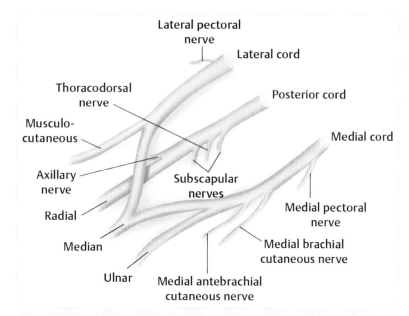

Fig. 4.17 Distal brachial plexus and branches. Aside from the major terminal branches, each cord has other smaller, "minor" branches: The lateral cord has one; both the medial and posterior cords have three.

4.3.2 Lateral Cord

The *lateral pectoral nerve* (C5, C6) originates from the proximal lateral cord, travels over the brachial plexus and axillary artery, pierces the clavipectoral fascia (which separates the pectoralis major from all other deep structures, including the pectoralis minor), and then fans out to innervate the *pectoralis major* from below. The lateral pectoral nerve concentrates its innervation upon the clavicular head of the pectoralis major. When this branch passes over the plexus, there is a reliable connection, or temporary merger, with the medial pectoral nerve, which, as the name implies, comes from the medial cord. The pectoralis major is a strong adductor and internal rotator of the arm. To test the clavicular head of the pectoralis major, and therefore the lateral pectoral nerve, have the patient abduct the arm 90 degrees with the elbow flexed and palm facing forward (▶ Fig. 4.18). Then, against resistance at the medial elbow, have the patient swing the arm toward midline. The lateral pectoral nerve is the only minor branch from the lateral cord.

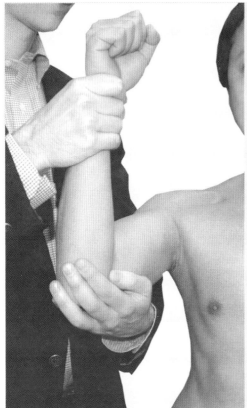

Fig. 4.18 Clavicular head of the pectoralis major (C5, C6) assessment: To test the clavicular head of the pectoralis major, start by having the patient abduct the arm 90 degrees with the elbow flexed. Then, against resistance at the medial elbow, instruct the patient to swing the arm anterior toward midline (across the chest).

4.3.3 Medial Cord

There are three minor branches from the medial cord: the more proximal medial pectoral nerve, and the more distal medial brachial and antebrachial cutaneous nerves. The *medial pectoral nerve* (C6–T1) innervates the *pectoralis minor*, which it passes through, and then pierces the clavipectoral fascia to innervate the sternal head of the *pectoralis major*. As mentioned, this nerve almost always communicates with the lateral pectoral nerve. To test the sternal head of the pectoralis major, the patient should begin with the elbow flexed 90 degrees and the arm abducted approximately 30 degrees. Instruct the patient to adduct the arm against resistance placed at the medial elbow (▸ Fig. 4.19). The pectoralis minor cannot be adequately isolated from the pectoralis major, and is therefore not assessed clinically.

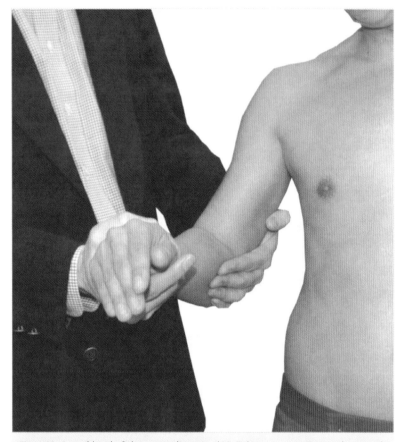

Fig. 4.19 Sternal head of the pectoralis major (C6, T1) assessment: To test the sternal head of the pectoralis major, the patient begins with the elbow flexed 90 degrees and the arm abducted approximately 30 degrees. Then instruct the patient to adduct the arm against resistance applied to the medial elbow.

Just prior to formation of the ulnar nerve, the medial cord gives off two branches: the *medial brachial cutaneous nerve* and the *medial antebrachial cutaneous nerve*. Both of these nerves were discussed in the ulnar nerve chapter because they are more readily understood in that context. In summary, sensory loss on the medial one half of the upper arm (medial brachial cutaneous) and forearm (medial antebrachial cutaneous) should be used to confirm involvement of the medial cord.

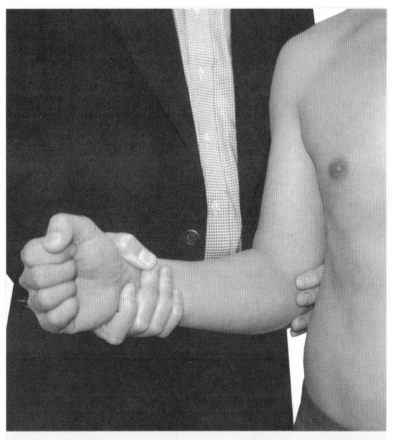

Fig. 4.20 Subscapularis (C5, C6) assessment: Have the patient internally rotate the arm while the elbow is flexed. Stabilize the elbow on the patient's side.

♦ The medial upper arm is part of the T2 dermatome. Therefore, the medial brachial cutaneous nerve returns sensation through the medial cord and lower trunk to the T2 spinal nerve. The presence of T2 axons in the brachial plexus has been excluded thus far for simplicity.

4.3.4 Posterior Cord

Like the medial cord, the posterior cord also has three minor branches. The muscles they innervate are easy to remember because they are the same three muscles that the radial nerve (terminal continuation of the posterior cord)

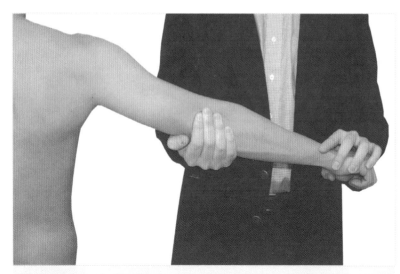

Fig. 4.21 Teres major (C5, C6) assessment: To test the teres major, begin with a straightened arm abducted horizontally with the palm down. Instruct the patient to adduct the arm against resistance while you inspect the teres major.

passes superficial to when exiting the axilla: the subscapularis, latissimus dorsi, and teres major. All three of these branches hang down like icicles from the posterior cord over the surface of the subscapularis muscle.

The first and last of these minor branches from the posterior cord are aptly named the *upper and lower subscapular nerves* (C5, C6). The upper subscapular nerve is not very long and enters the *subscapularis muscle* to innervate it. The subscapularis muscle (along with the teres major, latissimus dorsi, and pectoralis major) internally rotates the arm. Although the subscapularis muscle cannot be completely isolated, one can still test internal arm rotation (▶ Fig. 4.20). The lower subscapular nerve innervates the lower half of the subscapularis muscle, as well as the teres major. The teres major, along with the latissimus dorsi and pectoralis major, are the main arm adductors. To test the teres major, begin with a straightened arm abducted horizontally with the palm down. Instruct the patient to adduct the extended arm against resistance while you inspect the teres major (▶ Fig. 4.21). The other minor branch from the posterior cord is the *thoracodorsal nerve,* which arises between the upper and lower subscapular nerves. The thoracodorsal nerve innervates the latissimus dorsi muscle. To assess the latissimus dorsi, the patient adducts the arm when the elbow is flexed 90 degrees (▶ Fig. 4.22). In summary, all of the branches from the posterior cord act to adduct and internally rotate the arm.

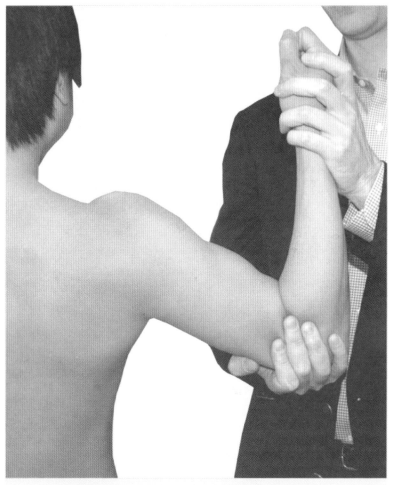

Fig. 4.22 Latissimus dorsi (C6–C8) assessment: To assess the latissimus dorsi, have the patient adduct the arm when the elbow is flexed 90 degrees.

4.4 Brachial Plexus Divisions and the Complete Picture

Chapters 1, 2, and 3 reviewed the median, ulnar, and radial nerves. This section discussed the remaining branches of the brachial plexus, including the

109

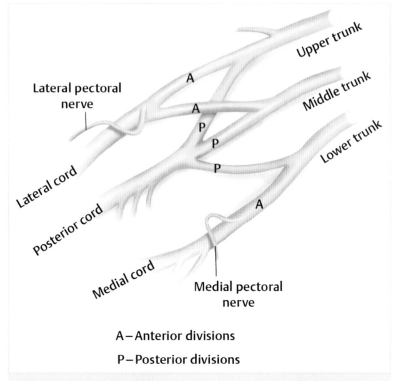

Lateral pectoral nerve

Upper trunk

Middle trunk

Lower trunk

A

A

P

P

P

A

Lateral cord

Posterior cord

Medial cord

Medial pectoral nerve

A – Anterior divisions

P – Posterior divisions

Fig. 4.23 Brachial plexus divisions. The posterior cord is formed by all three posterior divisions, the lateral cord from the anterior divisions of the upper and middle trunks, and the medial cord from the lower trunk's anterior division.

musculocutaneous and axillary nerves, as well as several "minor" branches. The hard part is over; connecting the proximal and distal ends of the plexus is easy.

The brachial plexus divisions connect the trunks to the cords (▶ Fig. 4.23). There are no distinct branches off the divisions. Each of the three trunks has both anterior and posterior divisions. All three posterior divisions merge to create the posterior cord. The anterior divisions from the upper and middle trunks create the lateral cord; only the anterior division of the lower trunk forms the medial cord. The posterior cord receives the largest number of divisions (three); this can be remembered by the fact that the posterior cord subsequently yields the largest terminal branch of the plexus, the radial nerve. The medial cord receives the anterior division of the lower trunk, which con-

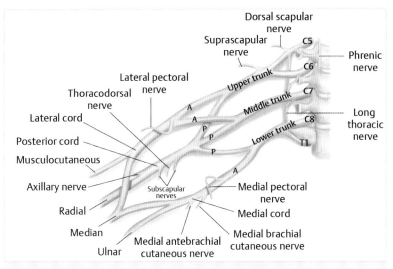

Fig. 4.24 The complete brachial plexus and its branches.

sists of the C8 and T1 spinal nerves. Knowing that the ulnar nerve is predominantly C8 and T1, it makes sense that the medial cord, which continues distally as the ulnar nerve, originates from the anterior division of the lower trunk (▶ Fig. 4.24).

♦ **The ulnar nerve can also have a C7 contribution. In this case, a more distal, accessory communication from the lateral cord to the ulnar nerve is usually present, which carries this C7 input.**

4.5 Regional Anatomical Relationships

The brachial plexus runs in a linear path from the intervertebral foramina, under the clavicle, through the axilla, finally ending in the medial arm. It is intimately associated with numerous muscular, arterial, and venous structures as it passes through these regions.

The proximal brachial plexus is located within the posterior triangle of the neck. This posterior triangle is defined by the sternocleidomastoid muscle anteriorly, the trapezius posteriorly, and the clavicle inferiorly. The posterior belly of the omohyoid traverses the lower aspect of the posterior triangle, converging with the suprascapular nerve at the scapula.

The brachial plexus passes through the interscalene triangle, which is defined by the anterior scalene, middle scalene, and first rib. The apex of the interscalene triangle is located in the posterior triangle of the neck. The anterior and middle scalenes originate from the anterior and posterior tubercles, respectively, of multiple cervical transverse processes. These muscles run down and attach along the first rib, with the spinal nerves and brachial plexus being sandwiched between them. The region where the brachial plexus and subclavian artery exit from between the scalenes and over the first rib is a potential site of entrapment (thoracic outlet syndrome). The brachial plexus divisions lie deep to the clavicle, whereas the cords and their branches are deep to the pectoralis minor and coracoid process. In the axilla, the brachial plexus cords lie between the clavipectoral fascia (superficial) and subscapularis muscle (deep).

The subclavian vessels exit the thorax via the ring of the first rib. The anterior scalene runs between the subclavian artery and vein, with the artery being posterior and adjacent to the C8, T1 spinal nerves and lower trunk. The vein is anterior to the anterior scalene, just deep to the clavicle. Originating from the subclavian artery soon after it emerges from the thorax, two small arterial branches traverse the posterior triangle of the neck over the brachial plexus. The more superior one is the transverse (superficial) cervical artery, and the lower one is the suprascapular artery. The latter joins the suprascapular nerve near the suprascapular notch. A third artery, called the dorsal scapular artery, often passes between the upper and middle trunks of the brachial plexus.

The blood supply to the proximal brachial plexus is from the subclavian system. Specifically, the vertebral and ascending cervical arteries supply C5 and C6, the deep cervical artery irrigates C7, and the superior intercostal arteries perfuse C8 and T1.

As expected, the venous anatomy surrounding the brachial plexus is variable. The subclavian vein runs anterior to the anterior scalene and receives the axillary vein, which runs medial and ventral to the axillary artery in the axilla. The posterior cord lies deep to these two veins. The external jugular vein drains into the subclavian vein under the clavicular attachment of the sternocleidomastoid. The external jugular vein, in general, begins at the angle of the jaw and runs toward the shoulder by crossing the lower, anterior aspect of the posterior triangle. It runs deep to the platysma, and occasionally deep to the posterior belly of the omohyoid.

4.6 The Cervical Plexus

The other plexus in the neck, the *cervical plexus,* originates from the C1 to C4 ventral rami. After emerging from their respective intervertebral foramina, these ventral rami merge and communicate with each other, ultimately yielding several deep (motor) and superficial (sensory) branches.

The deep branches innervate various muscles in the neck (scalenes, strap muscles, levator scapula, etc.). The *ansa cervicalis* innervates the strap muscles of the neck and is derived from these deep motor branches. The superior loop of the ansa cervicalis is composed of C1 and C2 ventral rami, whereas the inferior loop is from C2 and C3. The superior and inferior loops of the ansa cervicalis join anterior to the jugular vein.

In contrast to the deep branches, the superficial branches of the cervical plexus pour over (around and superficial to) the posterior edge of the sternocleidomastoid muscle to provide sensory coverage from the neck down to the shoulder and upper chest, including the area just below the clavicle (▶ Fig. 4.25). Four named sensory branches originate from the cervical plexus, from superior to inferior: the lesser occipital, greater auricular, transverse cervical, and supraclavicular nerves (▶ Fig. 4.26). If one follows the great auricular nerve back to the point where it emerges from below the sternocleidomastoid muscle, the spinal accessory nerve can often be located just a few millimeters more cranial (and deep) to this point. The only nerve from the cervical plexus that crosses the posterior triangle of the neck is the supraclavicular nerve and its terminal branches.

- The greater occipital nerve originates from the *dorsal* ramus of C2.
- C1 provides no sensation to the skin.
- The spinal accessory nerve (CN XI) crosses the most cranial aspect of the neck's posterior triangle.

4.7 Spinal Accessory Nerve (CN XI)

The *spinal accessory nerve* consists of intraspinal branches from C1 to C4, along with branches from the medulla. These branches merge intradurally, with the spinal accessory nerve, once formed, exiting the skull base via the jugular foramen. Its relationship to the jugular vein just below the skull base is variable. After the spinal accessory nerve innervates the sternocleidomastoid muscle, which is also innervated by deep motor branches of the cervical plexus, it exits from below the sternocleidomastoid and enters the posterior triangle of the neck, approximately 8 cm superior to the clavicle. The spinal accessory nerve travels toward the top of the shoulder, eventually passing under the trapezius muscle, which it innervates (▶ Fig. 4.26). As mentioned previously, this nerve commonly emerges from under the sternocleidomastoid muscle just cranial to the greater auricular nerve, the latter being an excellent surgical landmark. Across the posterior triangle, the spinal accessory nerve is interwoven with a major chain of lymph nodes.

The most common cause of isolated spinal accessory nerve palsy is iatrogenic injury following cervical lymph node dissection or biopsy. A painful, idiopathic neuropathy may also affect this nerve, which is thought to be a variant of acute brachial plexitis. *Vernet syndrome* consists of spinal accessory, vagus, and glossopharyngeal damage at the jugular foramen, through which all three

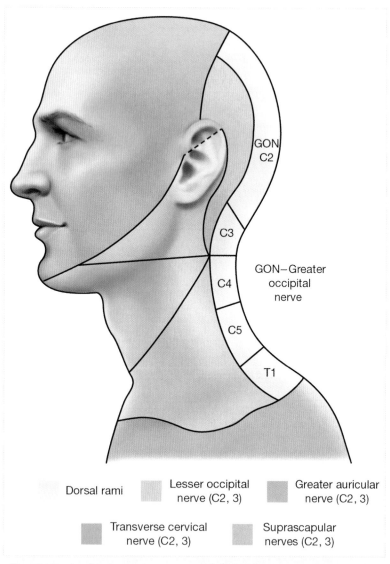

Fig. 4.25 Head and neck sensory coverage, excluding the face. Sensory branches from the cervical plexus, along with the dorsal rami of the upper cervical spinal nerves, provide innervation to this area. Of note, the greater occipital nerve originates solely from the dorsal rami of C2 and is not considered a branch of the cervical plexus.

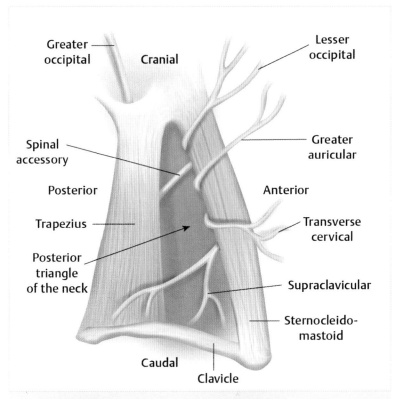

Fig. 4.26 Cervical plexus and spinal accessory nerve (schematic). Four named sensory branches originate from the cervical plexus, from superior to inferior: the lesser occipital, greater auricular, transverse cervical, and supraclavicular. The only sensory nerve from the cervical plexus that crosses the posterior triangle of the neck is the supraclavicular nerve. The spinal accessory nerve emerges from under the sternocleidomastoid just a few millimeters cranial to the greater auricular nerve.

of these nerves pass. This syndrome is usually from a local metastatic deposit or schwannoma.

Spinal accessory nerve palsy causes trapezial weakness. A patient with a weak trapezius will report trouble abducting the arm above the head (laterally), as well as shoulder girdle discomfort. This is because the trapezius assists the deltoid in abducting the arm above 90 degrees. Discomfort is thought to be from stress to muscles and ligaments that compensate for the trapezial weakness. At rest, the affected shoulder often lies lower than the unaffected one. Even with a complete trapezial palsy, shoulder shrug weakness seldom occurs. This is because the levator scapula also shrugs the shoulder (innervated by C3 and C4 via the cervical plexus). Weakness of the sternocleidomastoid muscle is rare, not only because the motor branches from the spinal accessory nerve branch quite proximally but also because this muscle receives coinnervation from the cervical plexus.

Secondary to the trapezial weakness, spinal accessory palsy also causes scapular winging. Trapezial winging is mild at rest and usually involves the upper border of the scapula, although this is variable. All types of winging (serratus anterior, trapezial, and rhomboid) are worse when the arm (partially flexed at the elbow) is pushed across the chest or in front of the body against resistance. However, only serratus anterior weakness causes winging when an extended, protracted arm is resisted. The presence of rhomboid weakness helps differentiate rhomboid versus trapezial winging. ▶ Table 4.1 compares the three muscular causes of scapular winging.

Table 4.1 Scapular winging: differential diagnosis

Nerve	Muscle	Scapular position at rest	Arm flexion at shoulder	Arm abduction at shoulder	Other
Long thoracic	Serratus anterior	Prominent inferomedial border	Causes winging		Winging when arm protracted
		Displaced medial	Difficulty > 60 degrees		
		Rotated downward			
Spinal accessory	Trapezius	Displaced lateral	Causes winging		Shoulder hangs lower
			Difficulty > 90 degrees		Trapezial atrophy
Dorsal scapular	Rhomboids	Prominent inferomedial border			Rhomboid weakness
		Displaced lateral			Rhomboid atrophy
		Rotated upward			

5 Clinical Evaluation of the Brachial Plexus

5.1 Proximal Brachial Plexus Palsies

5.1.1 Spinal Nerve Myotomes

Like spinal nerve dermatomes, spinal nerve myotomes are *approximate*. Nevertheless, learning spinal nerve myotomes is important for the clinical evaluation of patients with both cervical radiculopathies and proximal brachial plexus lesions. The C5 to T1 spinal nerve myotomes are presented here.

C5 Spinal Nerve: Arm Raise

The C5 spinal nerve's semiautonomous muscular innervation includes arm abduction and external rotation. These two movements are important for upper extremity function and are characteristically affected by upper brachial plexus injuries (e.g., birth palsy). The terminal branches mediating these movements include the axillary nerve to the deltoid muscle, and the suprascapular nerve to the supraspinatus and infraspinatus muscles. The supraspinatus (first 30 degrees) and deltoid (30–90 degrees) abduct the arm; the infraspinatus is the arm's most important external rotator (the teres major also externally rotates the arm). A composite movement involving all three of these muscles, and therefore predominantly mediated by the C5 nerve root, is the arm raise. Beginning with the arms straight along the side of the body, the patient abducts them to 90 degrees, while simultaneously externally rotating them so that the undersurface of the upper arm faces forward (▶ Fig. 5.1).

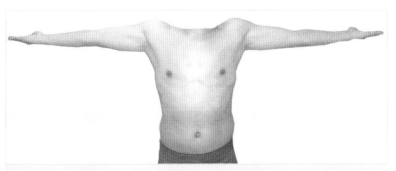

Fig. 5.1 Semiautonomous motor innervation of the C5 spinal nerve: the arm raise. Beginning with the arms straight along the side of the body, the patient simultaneously abducts and externally rotates the arms to 90 degrees.

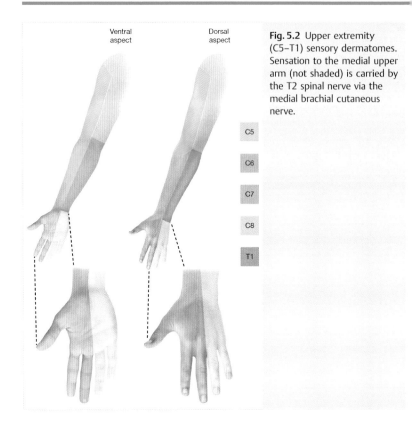

Ventral aspect

Dorsal aspect

C5

C6

C7

C8

T1

Fig. 5.2 Upper extremity (C5–T1) sensory dermatomes. Sensation to the medial upper arm (not shaded) is carried by the T2 spinal nerve via the medial brachial cutaneous nerve.

The C5 dermatome covers the lateral portion of the shoulder and upper arm down to the elbow (**F** Fig. 5.2). In part, the upper-lateral cutaneous nerve to the axillary nerve, as well as the lower-lateral brachial cutaneous nerve to the proximal radial nerve, carries sensation from this area.

C6 Spinal Nerve: Chin-Up

The C6 spinal nerve's semiautonomous muscular innervation includes forearm supination and elbow flexion, as well as extension and adduction of the arm at the shoulder. The radial nerve carries C6 innervation to the supinator (supination) and brachioradialis (elbow flexion with the forearm partially supinated). The musculocutaneous nerve carries fibers to the biceps brachii (elbow flexion and forearm supination) and brachialis (elbow flexion). The latissimus dorsi extends and adducts the arm at the shoulder via the thoracodorsal nerve, a movement that is primarily C6 mediated (C7 also provides significant innervation to the latissimus dorsi). A composite C6 movement would be the classic underhand chin-up. For this movement, the supinated forearm flexes at the elbow, and the latissimus dorsi contracts, pulling one's chin over the bar (▶ Fig. 5.3). With loss of C6 motor innervation the biceps and brachioradialis reflexes should be absent.

The lateral forearm and thumb are the sensory territory of the C6 spinal nerve (see ▶ Fig. 5.2). This sensation is carried in part by the lateral antebrachial cutaneous nerve to the musculocutaneous nerve, and for the thumb, by the terminal sensory branches of both the median and the radial nerves.

5.1.2 Upper Trunk

The upper trunk carries axons from the C5 and C6 spinal nerves. Traction injury to the upper trunk occurs when the shoulder is forced downward while the head is simultaneously stabilized or pushed in the opposite direction. This stretches the upper portion of the brachial plexus. It occurs with motorcycle trauma, falls, and birth palsies. An upper trunk injury is an *Erb palsy*. With this injury, the C5- and C6-innervated muscles are weak. The affected limb assumes a characteristic position at rest secondary to the unopposed action of the remaining musculature. The arm is adducted and internally rotated (unopposed pull of the pectoralis major), the elbow extended and the forearm pronated (unopposed pull of the triceps and pronator teres), and the wrist and fingers flexed (from weak finger and wrist extensors [variable C6 innervation]). It is called the *waiter's tip position* (▶ Fig. 5.4).

Similar mechanisms of injury may cause either an upper trunk or a spinal nerve injury. However, weakness involving the rhomboids (dorsal scapular nerve), serratus anterior (long thoracic nerve), and/or diaphragm (phrenic nerve), helps localize the injury to the C5 and C6 spinal nerves, where these branches originate, rather than the upper trunk per se. A lesion involving the upper trunk, or alternatively both the C5 and C6 spinal nerves, causes sensory loss on the lateral half of the arm and forearm, as well as the whole thumb (▶ Fig. 5.5).

5.1.3 Middle Trunk

C7 Spinal Nerve: Triceps Pushdown

The middle trunk is composed of fibers from only the C7 spinal nerve; hence they will be considered together. The C7 nerve's semiautonomous muscular control includes the triceps (radial nerve), flexor carpi radialis (median nerve), flexor carpi ulnaris (ulnar nerve), and pronator teres (median nerve). C7 also provides innervation to the wrist extensors, finger extensors, and finger flexors; however, this is either variable or strongly shared with other nerve roots (e.g., C6, C8). Therefore, wrist extension and finger extension/flexion are not

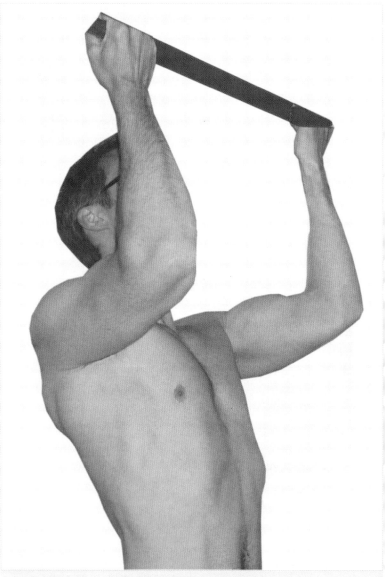

Fig. 5.3 Semiautonomous motor innervation of the C6 spinal nerve: the chin-up. For this movement the supinated forearm flexes at the elbow and the latissimus dorsi contracts; this pulls the chin over the bar.

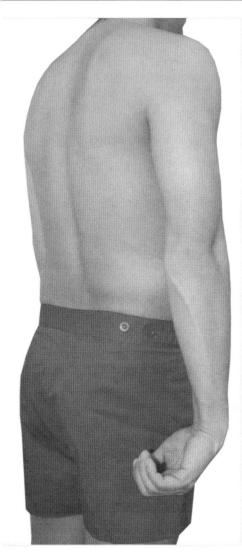

Fig. 5.4 Erb palsy or waiter's tip position (simulated). Patients characteristically have the affected arm adducted and internally rotated (unopposed pull of the pectoralis major), the elbow extended and forearm pronated (unopposed pull of the triceps and pronator teres), and the wrist and fingers flexed (from weak finger and wrist extensors [variable C6 innervation]).

considered autonomous to C7. The composite movement of the C7 spinal nerve or middle trunk is the triceps pushdown. This movement is made, for example, when you push down on a tabletop when getting up from being seated (▶ Fig. 5.6). For this to occur, one places the forearms in pronation (pronator teres), flexes the wrists (flexor carpi radialis and ulnaris), and contracts the

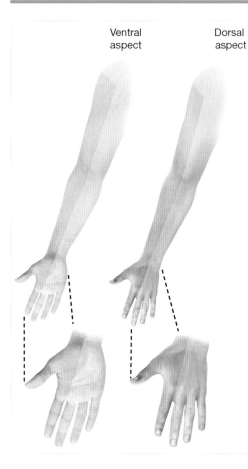

Ventral aspect

Dorsal aspect

Fig. 5.5 Sensory loss for an upper trunk or combination C5/C6 spinal nerve injury. This lesion yields a sensory loss involving the lateral half of the arm and forearm, as well as the whole thumb.

triceps to extend the elbows. A person with a middle trunk palsy cannot do this. It is not possible to differentiate a middle trunk from a C7 spinal nerve lesion based on motor examination alone. To do so, one must use other clinical and radiographic findings (e.g., evidence of rootlet avulsion on magnetic resonance imaging or myelography, paraspinal muscle denervation on electromyography, spinal nerve lesions present at adjacent levels, etc.).

The volar and dorsal aspects of the long finger are almost exclusively within the C7 dermatome (see ▶ Fig. 5.2). The sensory division of the median nerve (volar aspect of the long finger and its nail bed) and the superficial sensory radial nerve (dorsal aspect of the long finger) carry this sensation. Lesions of the middle trunk, consisting solely of C7 fibers, logically have the same pattern of sensory loss.

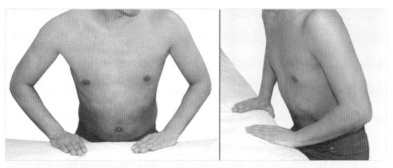

Fig. 5.6 Semiautonomous motor innervation of the C7 spinal nerve: triceps pressdown. This movement is made when you push down on a tabletop when getting up. For this to occur, one places the forearm in pronation (pronator teres), flexes the wrist (flexor carpi radialis), and contracts the triceps to extend the elbow.

C8 Spinal Nerve: Hand Grasp

The C8 spinal nerve provides motor input to many of the long finger flexors (and extensors), as well as to the hand intrinsic muscles. Innervation of the hand intrinsics is shared with T1. Some common muscles that are weak with a C8 palsy include the flexor profundi to the index and long finger (distal interphalangeal joint flexion), thenar intrinsics including the abductor pollicis brevis and opponens pollicis, and extensors to the thumb, forefinger, and long finger. Therefore, an easy way to assess C8 function is to have the patient grasp *and let go*, especially with the first three digits (▶ Fig. 5.7). A C8 palsy would prevent the patient from performing this movement.

The C8 dermatome covers the medial (i.e., ulnar) third of the hand, including the fifth digit and lateral hypothenar eminence (see ▶ Fig. 5.2). The dorsal ulnar cutaneous and palmar ulnar cutaneous nerves, along with the superficial sensory division of the ulnar nerve, carry sensation from this area.

T1 Spinal Nerve: Spreading the Fingers

The T1 spinal nerve is evaluated in near isolation by having the patient spread the fingers (▶ Fig. 5.8). This movement is mediated by the dorsal interossei muscles, which are predominantly T1 innervated. Atrophy of the first dorsal interosseous muscle, when present, is readily observed. The ulnar nerve carries T1 motor fibers to the dorsal interossei muscles. The T1 sensory dermatome covers the medial half of the forearm (see ▶ Fig. 5.2), with its sensory fibers carried by the medial antebrachial cutaneous nerve, a distal branch of the medial cord.

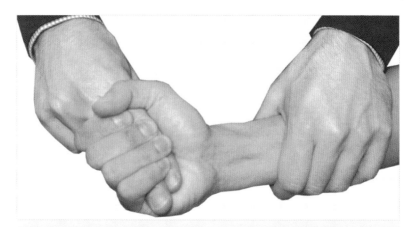

Fig. 5.7 Semiautonomous motor innervation of the C8 spinal nerve: hand grasp. A quick and easy way to assess C8 function is to have the patient grasp *and let go*, especially with the first three digits. Patients with C8 palsies have trouble doing this smoothly, strongly, and repetitively.

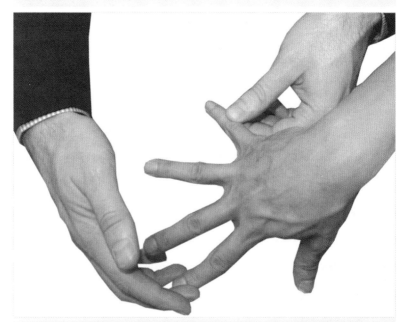

Fig. 5.8 Semiautonomous motor innervation of the T1 spinal nerve: spreading the fingers. The T1 spinal nerve is best tested in isolation by having the patient spread the fingers. The dorsal interossei muscles control this movement. Atrophy of the first dorsal interosseous muscle, when present, is readily observed.

5.1.4 Lower Trunk

Because the lower trunk comprises the C8 and T1 spinal nerves, injuries of the lower trunk cause marked hand weakness, including problems with hand grasp and finger spreading. Patients with lower trunk injuries should have good shoulder and elbow function, but report trouble with fine finger movements and grip strength. A lower trunk (or combination C8 and T1 spinal nerve) palsy causes sensory loss along the medial portion of the forearm and hand, including the fifth digit (▶ Fig. 5.9).

Injury to both the C8 and T1 spinal nerves is a *Klumpke palsy.* This injury may occur from a sudden upward pull of a child's outstretched arm, or following an injury where the extremity is suddenly forced upward (e.g., grasping an

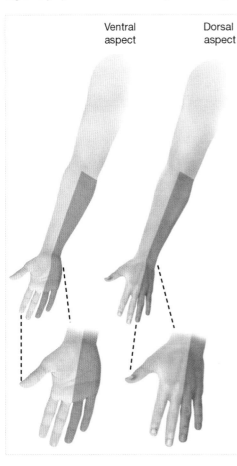

Ventral aspect

Dorsal aspect

Fig. 5.9 Sensory loss for a lower trunk or C8, T1 spinal nerve lesion. This lesion causes a sensory loss in the medial portion of the forearm and hand, including the fifth digit.

edge when falling, motorcycle accidents). Birth palsy may rarely present as an isolated Klumpke palsy.

Pancoast syndrome refers to the invasion and compression of the lower trunk by an apical lung mass. It usually begins with pain radiating down the inner aspect of the arm and forearm. Approximately one third of patients develop motor and sensory deficits, and two thirds have Horner syndrome. Small tumors can be undetectable on X-ray; therefore, a computed tomographic scan or magnetic resonance imaging with contrast is often required to confirm the diagnosis.

♦ **The medial upper arm is predominantly covered by the T2 dermatome. The T3 dermatome includes the axilla and a portion of the proximal, medial upper arm.**

5.1.5 Summary

Understanding the spinal nerve myotomes is required to assess proximal brachial plexus injuries. Patterns of muscular weakness are used to localize the injury to one or more of the spinal nerves or trunks. Sensory loss of the upper lateral arm (C5), thumb (C6), long finger (C7), fifth finger (C8), and medial forearm (T1) is then used to confirm your localization. Muscles innervated by branches directly off the spinal nerves or upper trunk (long thoracic, phrenic, dorsal scapular, and suprascapular nerves) may be examined and used to further localize the lesion. Pseudomeningoceles observed on radiographic imaging, as well as certain findings on electrodiagnostic tests, help confirm direct involvement of the spinal nerves (to be described).

5.2 Distal Brachial Plexus Palsies

5.2.1 Plus Palsies

The easiest way to remember the clinical manifestations of a cord lesion is to think of what happens to a patient with a musculocutaneous, ulnar, or radial nerve palsy (the terminal branches of each cord), and then add to these nerves' respective patterns of weakness any muscles innervated by other branches from the cord in question. I call these *plus palsies.*

5.2.2 Lateral Cord: Musculocutaneous Plus Palsy

The lateral cord is formed by the anterior divisions of both upper and middle trunks, and therefore, contains fibers from C5, C6, and C7. This cord bifurcates to provide the median nerve's lateral component (C5 to C7), and then continues distally as the musculocutaneous nerve. As expected, an isolated lesion to the lateral cord consists of a musculocutaneous nerve palsy, *plus* a partial median nerve deficit; that is, a deficit involving only the median nerve's C5 to C7 portion. This deficit may be termed a musculocutaneous *plus* palsy (▶ Fig. 5.10).

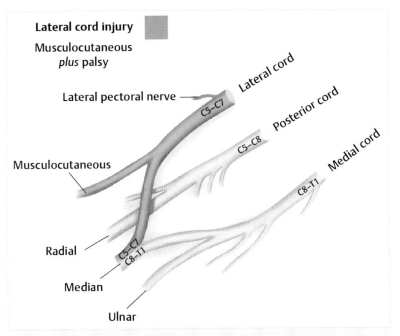

Fig. 5.10 Musculocutaneous plus palsy (lateral cord injury). The lateral cord terminates as the median nerve's lateral component (C5–C7) and musculocutaneous nerve. As expected, an isolated lesion to the lateral cord consists of a musculocutaneous nerve palsy plus a partial median nerve deficit involving its C5 to C7 portion.

The classic musculocutaneous palsy causes elbow flexion weakness secondary to biceps brachii, coracobrachialis, and brachialis weakness, and sensory loss in the lateral forearm (lateral antebrachial cutaneous nerve). As mentioned, median nerve function can be divided into lateral (C5–C7; lateral cord) and medial (C8, T1; medial cord) components. The lateral cord provides all the median nerve's sensory fibers (the medial cord does not provide cutaneous sensation to the median nerve). Therefore, lateral palm and first three digit sensory loss occurs with a lateral cord injury. Although the lateral component is primarily sensory, it also controls some proximal median nerve–innervated muscles (pronator teres and flexor carpi radialis). In contrast, the medial (C8, T1) component controls the distal median nerve–innervated muscles (hand intrinsics). The long finger flexors (flexor digitorum superficialis and the flexor digitorum profundus to the first two fingers) represent an intermediate gray zone, with contribution from both median nerve components. However, the C8 and T1 contribution is usually greater for these muscles.

127

Therefore, a lateral cord injury causes a musculocutaneous palsy (elbow flexion weakness), *plus* forearm pronation and wrist flexion weakness secondary to involvement of the lateral cord's motor contribution to the median nerve. Sensory loss in the lateral forearm and tips of the first three digits should also be present following a lateral cord injury. Furthermore, weakness of the clavicular head of the pectoralis major should occur, considering that the lateral pectoral nerve, which innervates this muscle, originates from the lateral cord.

5.2.3 Medial Cord: Ulnar Plus Palsy

The medial cord is a continuation of the lower trunk's anterior division, containing C8 and T1 nerve fibers. Although an accessory branch from the lateral cord donating some C7 fibers can occur, this is omitted for simplicity. The medial cord provides the medial component of the median nerve, containing C8 and T1 fibers, and then continues as the ulnar nerve into the arm. Therefore, an isolated medial cord lesion consists of an ulnar nerve palsy, *plus* the loss of C8, T1 median nerve function (▶ Fig. 5.11).

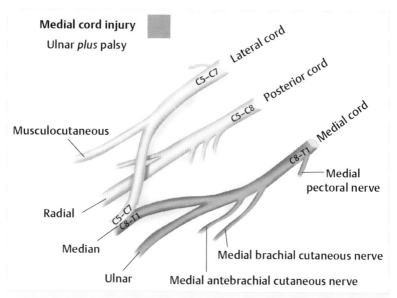

Fig. 5.11 Ulnar plus palsy (medial cord injury). The medial cord provides the medial contribution to the median nerve, containing C8 and T1 fibers, and then continues as the ulnar nerve into the arm. Therefore, an isolated medial cord lesion consists of an ulnar nerve palsy plus weakness in the muscles controlled by the C8 and T1 components of the median nerve.

An ulnar palsy causes weakness in medial wrist flexion (flexor carpi ulnaris), distal interphalangeal joint flexion weakness involving the fourth and fifth digits (flexor digitorum profundus), other fifth digit movements (opponens, flexor, and abductor digiti minimi), and finger abduction and adduction (interossei). Ulnar nerve sensory loss involves the medial third of the hand. As mentioned, the medial component of the median nerve controls the median nerve–innervated hand intrinsics, including the opponens pollicis, flexor pollicis brevis (superficial head), abductor pollicis brevis, and the first two lumbricals. Therefore, a medial cord lesion, or ulnar *plus* palsy, would, in addition to causing ulnar motor loss, cause median nerve–innervated thumb weakness, as well as difficulty extending the proximal interphalangeal joints of the first two fingers (lumbricals). Of note, these C8, T1 median nerve muscles are the same ones whose innervation is exchanged with a Martin-Gruber anastomosis (see Chapter 1).

The medial cord has a few side branches that can be tested to confirm its involvement. The medial brachial and antebrachial cutaneous nerves originate from the distal medial cord and carry sensation from the medial aspect of the arm and forearm, respectively. The medial pectoral nerve originates from the proximal medial cord, and, if damaged, causes weakness in the sternal head of the pectoralis major.

5.2.4 Posterior Cord: Radial Plus Palsy

The posterior cord is made up of the posterior division of all three trunks, containing input from C5 to C8. The presence of T1 fibers in the posterior cord is controversial and, needless to say, variable. The terminal branches of the posterior cord are the radial and axillary nerves; therefore, a combination palsy of these two nerves is the hallmark of a posterior cord injury (▶ Fig. 5.12). Hence, a posterior cord injury may be called a radial-axillary palsy or radial *plus* palsy.

A radial palsy causes weakness in elbow extension (triceps), forearm supination (supinator), wrist extension (extensor carpi radialis longus and brevis, extensor carpi ulnaris), and finger/thumb extension (superficial and deep finger extensors). Radial nerve sensory loss involves the posterior arm (posterior brachial cutaneous nerve) and forearm (posterior antebrachial cutaneous nerve), the lower lateral aspect of the arm (lower lateral brachial cutaneous nerve), and the dorsolateral hand (superficial sensory radial nerve). An axillary palsy causes arm abduction weakness secondary to deltoid paralysis. An axillary nerve lesion can also cause sensory loss in the upper lateral arm (upper lateral brachial cutaneous nerve). Furthermore, arm adduction and internal rotation weakness helps confirm posterior cord damage because branches off the posterior cord control these movements (i.e., the upper and lower subscapular and the thoracodorsal nerves).

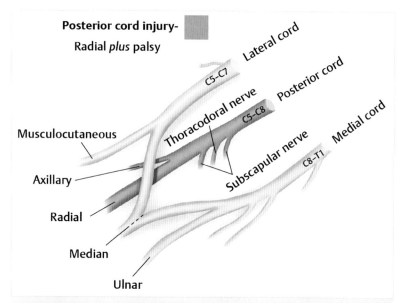

Fig. 5.12 Radial plus palsy (radial-axillary palsy, posterior cord injury). The two terminal branches of the posterior cord are the radial and axillary nerves; therefore, a palsy affecting these two nerves is the hallmark of a posterior cord injury.

5.2.5 Summary

To assess the distal brachial plexus, one needs to be familiar with patterns of neurological deficits that may occur following injury to its terminal branches: the musculocutaneous, median, ulnar, radial, and axillary nerves. With this knowledge, diagnosis of cord-level injuries becomes straightforward; cord injuries cause deficits that are a combination of those seen with injury to their branches. Therefore, analogous to proximal brachial plexus injury being assessed by referring to its spinal nerve components, the distal plexus is evaluated by using knowledge of its major terminal branches.

5.3 Assessment of Divisional Injuries

Isolated injury to one of the brachial plexus divisions can be difficult to differentiate clinically from cord or trunk lesions. Therefore, it is usually not possible to say if the divisions are damaged in addition to cords or trunks without surgical exploration.

An isolated injury to one, or more, divisions yields neurological deficits that are the same, or less severe, than a cord-level injury. For example, an injury to the anterior division of the lower trunk (C8, T1) should involve nearly all the fibers in the medial cord. However, a divisional injury affecting the lateral cord may involve only the anterior division from the upper trunk (C5, C6) or the anterior division from the middle trunk (C7). Injury to any of the three posterior divisions will cause a partial posterior cord deficit. For instance, an isolated injury to the posterior division of the upper trunk may be confused with an axillary nerve palsy; however, the presence of some brachioradialis and supinator weakness, along with sensory loss on the dorsal thumb (C6 dermatome via superficial sensory radial nerve) should point to a partial cord or divisional injury rather than an axillary nerve palsy.

With an ability to readily diagnose proximal and distal brachial plexus lesions, one can deduce a divisional injury. Nevertheless divisional lesions may be indistinguishable from partial cord injuries. Fortunately, injuries involving only the divisions are infrequent.

5.4 Diagnosis of Preganglionic Injury

Stretch injuries to the brachial plexus can cause avulsion of the ventral and dorsal rootlets from the spinal cord itself. The C8 and T1 spinal rootlets are most prone to this type of injury because these spinal nerves have minimal anchoring to their respective troughs along the transverse processes. In contrast, the C5 to C6 spinal nerves are strongly attached to their respective transverse processes, thereby making avulsion at these levels less likely when a similar force is applied. There are multiple ways to determine if a spinal root has a preganglionic, or avulsion, injury, which is important for prognosis and treatment.

Myelography supplemented with postmyelography computed tomographic scanning has good sensitivity in detecting pseudomeningoceles and absent (avulsed) nerve rootlets at each cervical level. These two findings are highly suggestive of rootlet avulsion. Magnetic resonance imaging can also be used to document these findings; however, the images may not be of adequate resolution in some cases. Involvement of very proximal branches of the brachial plexus, including the phrenic nerve (paralyzed hemidiaphragm), dorsal scapular nerve (rhomboid weakness), and long thoracic nerve (scapular winging) also suggests preganglionic damage, or at least intraforaminal damage. Avulsion of the T1 spinal nerve can cause Horner syndrome, the presence of which should be readily apparent on examination.

Electrophysiological testing can help confirm preganglionic damage. With this type of injury, the peripheral nerve sensory axons remain connected to their cell bodies in the spinal ganglia. Therefore, the amplitudes of distal extremity sensory nerve action potentials remain normal (or increased), despite no sensation being present on examination. The presence of compound motor action potentials argues against spinal cord avulsion. Paraspinal denervation is also indicative of preganglionic or intraforaminal nerve injury.

5.5 Examination Approach

5.5.1 Comprehensive Examination

When examining the brachial plexus and upper extremity, one should employ a systematic approach, beginning proximal and proceeding distal. With the exception of a screening assessment in the emergency department, an abbreviated or focused examination is not recommended. This is because subtle, yet important, deficits can be missed. My examination routine is divided into six distinct steps (See Box: Six steps of a comprehensive brachial plexus examination (p. 132).

Six steps of a comprehensive brachial plexus examination

Back
- Observation
- Rhomboids
- Latissimus dorsi
- Trapezius
- Scapular winging

Shoulder
- Supraspinatus
- Deltoid
- Posterior deltoid
- Teres major
- Pectoralis major
- Infraspinatus

Arm
- Triceps
- Biceps
- Brachioradialis

Forearm
- Supinator
- Pronator
- Wrist flexion
- Wrist extension
- Finger extension

Hand
- Observation
- Finger flexion

- Thenar intrinsics
- Hypothenar intrinsics
- Interossei
- Lumbricals

Skin
- Sensation
- Perspiration/Horner syndrome
- Pulses/masses
- Reflexes/Tinel sign

- *Step 1: Back.* The exam begins with the patient facing away from the examiner. The presence at rest of scapular winging, muscle atrophy, and asymmetry of the shoulders and scapulae are noted. Next, the patient shrugs the shoulders upward to allow assessment of trapezial and levator scapulae function. Having the patient bring the scapulae together allows assessment of the rhomboids. The latissimus dorsi are palpated bilaterally, and the patient is asked to cough, which causes their contraction. The patient is instructed to raise the arms to the side and straight above the head to check trapezial function. Next, the patient is told to reach toward the wall with the affected arm, and scapular winging is evaluated.
- *Step 2: Shoulder.* Starting with the arm straight and to the side, the patient is instructed to abduct the arm. In doing so, the supraspinatus and deltoid are assessed. With the arm horizontal to the floor, the posterior head of the deltoid (posterior movement) and teres major (downward movement) are tested. The patient then flexes the forearm 90 degrees ("hold-up" position), and both the clavicular (lateral pectoral nerve) and sternal (medial pectoral nerve) heads of the pectoralis major are assessed, both visually and by palpation. Facing the patient's flank, external arm rotation is subsequently tested (infraspinatus).
- *Step 3: Arm.* The triceps are examined with the upper arm parallel to the floor, so the effect of gravity is eliminated. Elbow flexion is tested with the forearm both fully supinated (biceps brachii) and half supinated (brachioradialis).
- *Step 4: Forearm.* Supination and pronation are tested with the elbow straight. Next, wrist movement is assessed. The patient flexes the wrist (flexor carpi radialis and ulnaris), and then the arm is pronated and the wrist extensors are tested (extensor carpi radialis longus and brevis and extensor carpi ulnaris). With the forearm placed on a flat surface, the long forearm finger extensors (extensor digitorum communis, extensor indicis, extensor digiti minimi, and extensor pollicis longus and brevis) are evaluated.

- *Step 5: Hand.* The hand is first observed at rest for signs of atrophy. The patient is then instructed to open and close the hand so that any evidence of contracture can be observed, if present (e.g., claw hand). Next, the thumb is evaluated further, including abduction, adduction, opposition, and flexion. Froment and "okay" signs are evaluated. Flexion at the proximal (flexor digitorum superficialis) and distal (flexor digitorum profundus) interphalangeal joints is assessed. Abduction and opposition of the fifth digit are evaluated, as well as any Wartenberg or palmaris brevis signs. Finger abduction (dorsal interossei), adduction (palmar interossei), and extension at the interphalangeal joints are tested (lumbricals).
- *Step 6: Skin.* Light touch and pinprick are tested from the shoulder down to the fingers. Testing is performed circumferentially on the arm, forearm, and hand. Fingertip testing is especially important, considering that the thumb, long finger, and fifth digit represent different dermatomes. Any abnormality or asymmetry between the upper extremities is evaluated further, including assessment of two-point discrimination and localization. Lack of sweating may be observed with an ophthalmoscope. The neck and axilla are palpated and observed for scars, masses, or a Tinel sign. To finish, pulses and reflexes (C6, C7) are tested.

Lesion localization is then performed using one's knowledge of peripheral nerve anatomy. The deficit may then be graded for comparison with subsequent assessments.

5.5.2 The Screening Examination

In certain situations (e.g., in the emergency department or trauma slot) an abbreviated screening examination for brachial plexus injury may be indicated. This emergent evaluation, however, is often limited by other injuries, including long-bone fractures, spine trauma, and patient confusion or stupor. This screening examination, or primary survey, evaluates nine muscles that have been selected because they each follow a separate path through the brachial plexus (▶ Table 5.1). These muscles include two shoulder, three arm, and four hand muscles.

This primary survey is performed with the patient supine or sitting. The following two shoulder muscles are tested: deltoid and infraspinatus. Next, the following arm muscles are tested: biceps, brachioradialis, and triceps. Finally, hand movements are tested, including the flexor carpi radialis, extensor indicis, abductor pollicis brevis, and dorsal interossei.

If the primary survey reveals a deficit, a secondary survey in the emergency department includes sensory and additional motor testing. The primary survey reveals if the lesion is proximal or distal. Proximal lesions are then tested using a spinal nerve template (which spinal nerves are affected?), whereas distal

Table 5.1 The brachial plexus screening examination

Shoulder		
	Deltoid	C5, upper trunk, posterior cord, axillary nerve
	Infraspinatus	C5, upper trunk, supra-scapular nerve
Arm		
	Biceps	C6, upper trunk, lateral cord, musculocutaneous nerve
	Brachioradialis	C6, upper trunk, posterior cord, radial nerve
	Triceps	C7, middle trunk, posterior cord, radial nerve
Hand		
	Flexor carpi radialis	C7, middle trunk, lateral cord, median nerve
	Extensor indicis	C8, lower trunk, posterior cord, radial nerve
	Abductor pollicis brevis	C8, lower trunk, medial cord, median nerve
	Dorsal interossei	T1, lower trunk, medial cord, ulnar nerve

Note: The nine muscles are assessed proximal to distal. Spinal nerve contributions are simplified.

brachial plexus injuries are assessed with a cord approach (which cords are affected, and to what extent?). To perform the secondary survey, think of all the muscles innervated by the injured element (as determined by the primary survey, e.g., upper trunk, medial cord) and then test them all from proximal to distal. A comprehensive examination (described previously) should always be performed; however, in many trauma patients, this is completed later when the patient is fully cooperative and more time is available.

5.6 Processes Affecting the Brachial Plexus

Brachial plexus injuries are usually traumatic, with stretch (including birth palsies), lacerations, gunshots, and blunt contusions being common mechanisms. Other, less frequent etiologies include compression by anomalous fibrous ridges on the scalene musculature (neurogenic thoracic outlet syndrome), delayed radiation damage, and acute brachial plexitis (Parsonage-Turner syndrome). Considering the patient's history and risk factors, an accurate etiological diagnosis can usually be made even before examination. Some specific causes of brachial plexus injury are discussed here.

5.6.1 Neurogenic Thoracic Outlet Syndrome

Symptoms of neurogenic thoracic outlet syndrome, or *Gilliatt-Sumner hand,* are caused by irritation to the C8 and T1 spinal nerves and/or the lower trunk. "Disputed," arterial, and venous forms of thoracic outlet syndrome are separate clinical entities and will not be commented on. The source of irritation for neurogenic thoracic outlet syndrome is localized to the scalene triangle. The scalene triangle is made up of the anterior scalene anteriorly, the middle scalene posteriorly, and the edge of the first rib inferiorly. The brachial plexus and subclavian artery pass through this triangle, but the subclavian vein does not. Irritation of the brachial plexus is often from an abnormal fibrous band, on or near these two scalene muscles. An elongated C7 transverse process or cervical rib may be present, both of which unfavorably reorient the scalene muscles, possibly leading to neural compression or irritation. The patient with classic neurogenic thoracic outlet syndrome has forward-drooping shoulders.

Manifestations of neurogenic thoracic outlet syndrome are usually localized to the C8 and T1 spinal nerves. Patients have progressive hand intrinsic weakness and atrophy. Sensory loss, when present, occurs on the medial aspect of the forearm, as well as on the medial third of the hand. Hand intrinsic weakness and atrophy are often more median than ulnar, whereas sensory loss is all ulnar (ulnar and medial antebrachial cutaneous nerves, both from the medial cord). Pain is uncommon, but a dull ache in the shoulder girdle or axilla can occur. Externally rotating the arm while abducting it above the head often precipitates or worsens symptoms after a minute or two in this position (Roos maneuver or elevated arm stress test). Loss of a radial pulse with this maneuver (Adson sign) may also occur. Both of these provocative tests, however, have a high rate of false-positives. A supraclavicular Tinel sign may be present. An apical lordotic cervical radiograph documents a cervical rib or elongated C7 transverse process, when present.

Care must be taken to differentiate thoracic outlet syndrome from C8 radiculopathy or ulnar compression at the elbow. Concurrent weakness in median (abductor pollicis brevis) as well as ulnar (abductor digiti minimi or the first dorsal interosseous) innervated muscles helps confirm a more proximal injury to the brachial plexus (i.e., neurogenic thoracic outlet, *not* carpal or cubital tunnel syndrome). No history of neck or radicular pain, along with the presence of both C8 and T1 sensory and motor changes, helps exclude a single-level radiculopathy.

5.6.2 Birth-Related Brachial Plexus Palsy

Newborns can have stretch injuries to their proximal brachial plexus during difficult deliveries, vaginal or otherwise. Heavy birth weight is considered a predisposing factor. The most common injury is an *Erb palsy*, where C5 and C6 (or the upper trunk) are damaged. As described previously for adults, an infant with an Erb palsy maintains the arm adducted, elbow extended, forearm pronated, and wrist flexed (waiter's tip position). Another type of birth injury is *Klumpke palsy*, with damage to the C8 and T1 nerve roots. Although this palsy can occur during a breech delivery, with the arm hyperabducted above the head, it most commonly occurs after a face-first delivery where the head is hyperextended. Infants with Klumpke palsy are not able to grasp with the hand. Other types of birth brachial plexus injury include complete plexal injury and an *Erb plus palsy*. An Erb plus palsy is an injury involving C5, C6, *plus C7.*

Klumpke palsy is the least common type of birth palsy. The prognosis of both Klumpke palsy and complete brachial plexus palsy are significantly worse than that for Erb palsy. The latter often recovers spontaneously in a few months.

Examining an infant is challenging. Neurological diagnosis of an obstetrical palsy relies greatly on observing the arm and hand position at rest, a lack of movement, and upper extremity asymmetry during play and crawling. It is important to perform a series of examinations over time. Radiographs may be used to rule out fractures or a hemidiaphragm (phrenic palsy). Electrodiagnosis should be first performed 4 to 6 weeks after injury, and then on a serial basis (approximately every 3 months) to assess recovery. As the child grows, the neurological examination becomes more structured, including various arm movements of functional importance.

5.6.3 Acute Brachial Plexitis (Parsonage-Turner Syndrome)

Acute brachial plexitis presents with marked shoulder pain that often radiates down the arm, up the neck, or toward the scapula. Its onset is usually sudden and lasts for hours to a few weeks. This syndrome occurs more often in males and can affect any age group. A common position of comfort is the arm adducted and elbow flexed, the so-called adduction-flexion sign of acute brachial plexitis. Neck movement and Valsalva maneuvers do not usually exacerbate the pain. Cervical imaging helps rule out radiculopathy from a herniated disk. Weakness is usually not present during the acute, painful phase of this syndrome; however, as the pain resolves, paralysis of certain brachial plexus–innervated musculature occurs. The degree of eventual weakness often correlates with the severity of the initial pain. Although any, or all, upper extremity and shoulder girdle muscles may be involved, the most common muscles affected include the deltoid, supraspinatus, and infraspinatus. This syndrome may occur bilaterally, especially subclinically (i.e., seen only with electrodiagnostic testing on one side). Sensory loss is classically absent or minimal during acute brachial plexitis, a finding that helps confirm the diagnosis. Plexitis is a self-limiting process, with approximately 90% of patients returning to near normal in up to 3 years. The etiology is uncertain. About half of the patients report an antecedent viral illness, which points toward an inflammatory cause. Some patients have mild to moderate shoulder trauma or overuse as an instigating factor. Others may have recently undergone a surgical procedure. Electrophysiology is helpful for both diagnosis and prognosis.

♦ **A rare autosomal-dominant form of acute brachial plexitis has been reported. These patients have repeated bouts of characteristic pain and weakness, often involving different nerves. Although these episodes often follow stressful events, including childbirth, strenuous exercise, and infection, the majority of cases have no identifiable trigger. This hereditary disease can also affect children.**

5.6.4 Radiation-induced Brachial Plexopathy

Plexitis may occur following radiation treatment for cancer, usually breast cancer. Radiation damage can occur at any time after exposure (on average 5 years), and usually causes painless sensory and motor deficits in either the upper trunk or entire plexus; sole involvement of the lower trunk is uncommon. Horner syndrome does not usually occur, and if it does, metastatic plexopathy or an apical lung metastasis should be investigated. If pain is severe, recurrent cancer is more likely. Local radiation-induced skin changes are a common finding in these patients, although not universal.

6 Sciatic Nerve

6.1 Anatomical Course

6.1.1 Buttock

The sciatic nerve is the predominant output from the sacral plexus, being made up of axons from the L4, L5, S1, S2, and S3 spinal nerves. After formation, the sciatic nerve exits the pelvis via the greater sciatic foramen inferior to the pyriformis muscle. The pyriformis muscle originates on the lateral intrapelvic surface of the sacrum and inserts on the superior tip of the femur's greater trochanter. This muscle has a triangular shape, with its base on the sacrum and its apex on the trochanter.

After exiting the pelvis, the sciatic nerve passes distally toward the midline of the thigh, underneath the gluteus maximus, and over a bed of five successive muscles that run perpendicular to its course. From proximal to distal, they are the following: superior gemelli, obturator internus, inferior gemelli, quadratus femoris, and adductor magnus. The sciatic nerve is protected by the large gluteus maximus, as well as by the ischial tuberosity, when one sits. The sciatic nerve remains posterior (dorsal) to the adductor magnus as it courses down the thigh (▶ Fig. 6.1). The first three muscles (superior gemelli, obturator internus, and inferior gemelli) attach to the greater trochanter. The quadratus femoris inserts into the lesser trochanter; the adductor magnus has a long insertion on the shaft of the femur.

The sciatic nerve is actually two nerves, the tibial and common peroneal, which are joined by a common epineurium from the pelvis to the lower third of the thigh, where they separate. The tibial nerve is medial and larger, being composed of axons from L4 to S3. The common peroneal nerve is lateral and smaller, composed of axons from L4 to S2, with a large contribution from the lumbosacral trunk.

Before forming the sciatic nerve, the spinal nerve's ventral rami split into anterior and posterior divisions, with the tibial nerve being composed of the anterior divisions and the common peroneal the posterior divisions. This orientation is opposite than expected because the tibial nerve innervates posterior compartment muscles, whereas the common peroneal nerve innervates anterior compartment ones.

Also exiting the pelvis via the greater sciatic notch under the pyriformis muscle, medial to the sciatic nerve, are the posterior cutaneous nerve to the thigh (the lesser sciatic nerve), the inferior gluteal nerve and vessels, and, most medially, the pudendal nerve and vessels. The superior gluteal nerve exits the greater sciatic foramen superior to the pyriformis. These nerves are discussed in Chapter 8 on the lumbosacral plexus.

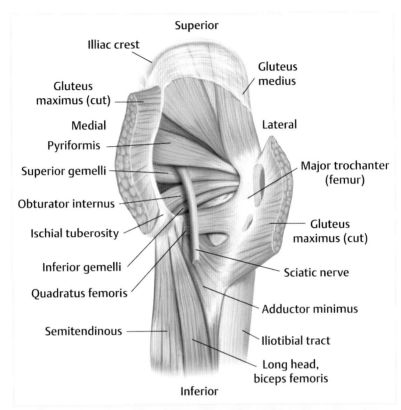

Fig. 6.1 The muscular anatomy of the piriformis and deep buttock muscles. After formation, the sciatic nerve exits the pelvis via the greater sciatic foramen inferior to the pyriformis muscle. Leaving the pelvis, the sciatic nerve runs distal toward the midline of the thigh, underneath the gluteus maximus and over a bed of five muscles that run perpendicular to its course.

♦ The sciatic nerve may also pass superior to, or even through, the pyriformis muscle when exiting the sciatic notch.
♦ The S3 contribution to the sciatic nerve is variable. Alternatively, the sciatic nerve sometimes contains axons from S4.

6.1.2 Thigh and Knee

The sciatic nerve passes down the midline of the posterior thigh toward the popliteal fossa. It runs superficial, or dorsal, to the adductor magnus, but underneath the hamstring muscles. There are four hamstring muscles, two medial and two lateral. The lateral two are the long and short heads of the biceps femoris. The long head of the biceps femoris originates from the ischial tuberosity; the short head originates from the shaft of the femur. Together, both heads insert distally into the fibular head. The long head of the biceps femoris crosses the midline of the thigh, similar to the arm of an X, from medial to lateral. The long head is superficial to the short head.

The medial pair of hamstrings are the semitendinous and semimembranous muscles, both originating from the ischial tuberosity and remaining medial along the thigh to insert into the lateral tibia, along with the sartorius and gracilis tendons. The semitendinous is more superficial and medial. The sciatic nerve runs deep to the hamstrings, mostly deep to the long head of the biceps femoris as this muscle passes medial to lateral. The sciatic nerve bifurcates into the tibial and common peroneal nerves approximately two thirds of the way down the thigh. Distally, like the archway of a door, both the medial and lateral groups of hamstrings separate from midline to expose the popliteal fossa.

The larger and more medial tibial nerve (anterior divisions of L4–S3) remains midline as it continues down the thigh and into the popliteal fossa. In the distal thigh, the tibial nerve joins the popliteal artery and vein. These vessels are the distal continuations of the femoral artery and vein, entering the posterior compartment of the thigh by passing medial to the femur via the adductor hiatus. Viewing the popliteal fossa from posterior, the tibial nerve lies lateral to the popliteal vessels (▶ Fig. 6.2). This neurovascular bundle runs deep into the lower leg (defined as the lower extremity between the knee and the ankle) by passing under the gastrocnemius and soleus muscles. Underneath these muscles, the tibial nerve runs over, or dorsal to, the popliteal muscle, which creates the floor of the popliteal fossa. The popliteal muscle passes transversely from the upper medial aspect of the tibia to the lower lateral femur.

Prior to entering the lower leg, the *medial sural cutaneous nerve* branches from the tibial nerve. This branch runs superficial along the midline between the two heads of the gastrocnemius muscle, eventually piercing the subcutaneous fascia. Upon piercing the fascia, the medial sural cutaneous nerve merges with the *lateral sural cutaneous nerve* (from the common peroneal nerve) to form the proper *sural nerve*. The sural nerve passes down the posterior lower leg, behind the lateral malleolus, and into the dorsolateral foot.

The common peroneal nerve (posterior divisions of L4–S2) runs obliquely from the apex of the popliteal fossa to the posterior fibular head (see ▶ Fig. 6.2). In doing so, this nerve skirts along the medial margin of the biceps femoris muscle. In this region, the common peroneal nerve gives off two sensory branches, the lateral sural cutaneous (mentioned earlier), which merges with the medial sural cutaneous (from the tibial nerve), and the *lateral cutaneous nerve to the calf*. After these two branches, the common peroneal nerve passes lateral to the proximal fibular shaft, underneath the peroneus longus muscle.

141

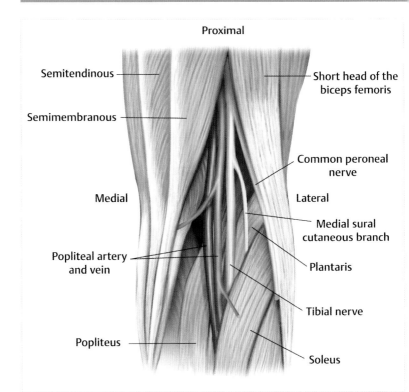

Fig. 6.2 Popliteal fossa anatomy. Viewing the popliteal fossa from posterior, the tibial nerve lies lateral to the popliteal artery and vein. The common peroneal nerve skirts along the medial margin of the biceps femoris muscle, from the apex of the popliteal fossa to the fibular head.

♦ The sural nerve is usually composed of both medial and lateral sural cutaneous nerves; however, in some patients the sural nerve is derived from only one of these two nerves, usually the medial one.

6.1.3 Tibial Nerve

Leg

The tibial nerve runs down the lower leg in a straight line from the middle of the popliteal fossa, to just posterior to the medial malleolus. This nerve runs deep to the gastrocnemius and soleus muscles but remains superficial (dorsal) to the deep posterior compartment muscles. In the proximal lower leg, the tibial nerve passes dorsal to the tibialis posterior muscle. In the distal lower leg it runs in a cleft between the flexor digitorum longus medially, and the flexor hallucis longus laterally. The popliteal artery and vein continue with the tibial nerve in the lower leg, but they are renamed the posterior tibial artery and vein. These vessels run on the nerve's medial aspect, first over the tibialis posterior, then over the flexor digitorum longus.

Posterior to the medial malleolus, the tibial nerve enters the foot by running deep to the flexor retinaculum (laciniate ligament). The flexor retinaculum is a thin ligament that bridges the medial malleolus to the calcaneus, under which passes not only the tibial nerve but also the posterior tibial artery and veins, and from anterior to posterior, the tendons of the tibialis posterior, flexor digitorum longus, and flexor hallucis longus. This subligamentous, anatomical passage into the foot is called the *tarsal tunnel* (▶ Fig. 6.3).

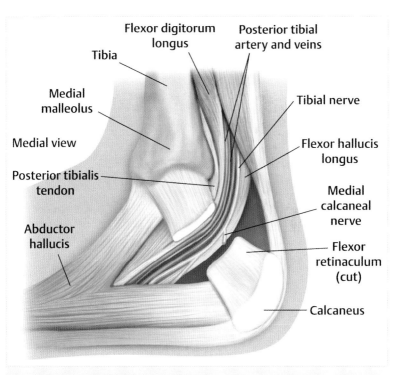

Fig. 6.3 The tarsal tunnel. Posterior to the medial malleolus, the tibial nerve enters the foot by running deep to the flexor retinaculum. The flexor retinaculum is a ligamentous band from the medial malleolus to the calcaneus, under which passes not only the tibial nerve but also the posterior tibial artery, veins, and multiple tendons.

Within, or just proximal to, the tarsal tunnel, the tibial nerve bifurcates into the medial and lateral plantar nerves. The tibial nerve also gives a sensory branch to the medial half of the heel just before, or from within, the tarsal tunnel. This branch is called the *medial calcaneal nerve.*

Foot

The medial plantar nerve is the larger of the two terminal divisions of the tibial nerve, and, as its name implies, it courses through the medial plantar region (▶ Fig. 6.4). The medial plantar nerve runs between the abductor hallucis and the flexor digitorum brevis, the latter muscle being located in the midline of the sole. As the medial plantar nerve passes through the foot, it splits into digital nerves for the first three and a half toes. In contrast, sensory branches to the sole originate quite proximally, just after the medial plantar nerve enters the sole of the foot.

After traversing the tarsal tunnel, the lateral plantar nerve passes across the sole of the foot, deep to the flexor digitorum brevis. Once lateral, it passes between the quadratus plantae medially and the abductor digiti minimi pedis laterally. The lateral plantar nerve divides into superficial sensory and deep motor branches, analogous to the ulnar nerve in the hand. The superficial branch becomes subcutaneous, whereas the deep branch remains deep to innervate the intrinsic foot musculature.

6.1.4 Common Peroneal Nerve

Deep Branch

The common peroneal nerve passes around the lateral aspect of the upper fibula, just distal to the fibular head, underneath the posterior fibrous edge of the peroneus longus muscle. Two ligamentous bands in this region form the so-called fibular tunnel: the peroneus longus muscle aponeurosis (deep) and an aponeurosis connecting the soleus and peroneal fascia (superficial). Under the peroneus longus, the common peroneal nerve bifurcates into a superficial and deep branch.

Anterior to the fibula, the deep peroneal nerve dives below the extensor digitorum longus muscle, where it joins the tibialis anterior artery to travel down the lower leg. This neurovascular bundle runs between the extensor digitorum longus anteriorly and the intermuscular septum/lateral tibia posteriorly. In the more distal aspect of the lower leg, the deep peroneal nerve shifts a little toward the midline, where it runs on the tibia under the tibialis anterior muscle. The deep peroneal nerve travels along the dorsal aspect of the foot by running under two extensor retinaculums (superior and inferior), which together create the *anterior tarsal tunnel.* Once on the dorsum of the foot, the

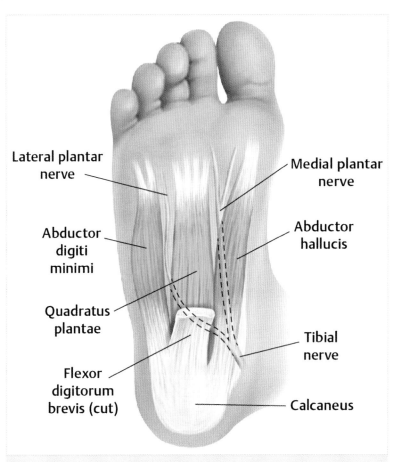

Fig. 6.4 Muscular relationships of the plantar nerves in the sole of the foot. The medial plantar nerve runs between the abductor hallucis and the flexor digitorum brevis, the latter muscle being located in the midline of the sole. The lateral plantar nerve passes across the sole of the foot, deep to the flexor digitorum brevis. Once lateral, it runs anteriorly between the quadratus plantae medially and the abductor digiti minimi pedis laterally.

deep peroneal nerve divides into medial and lateral branches. The medial branch passes distally with the dorsalis pedis artery, eventually terminating as a sensory branch to the first web space. The lateral branch innervates the extensor digitorum brevis.

145

Superficial Branch

The superficial branch of the common peroneal nerve turns distal after passing around the fibula to run under the peroneus longus. It, however, remains superficial to the extensor digitorum longus. This latter muscle separates the superficial and deep branches of the peroneal nerve. The superficial branch emerges in the distal half of the lower leg, lateral to the formed tendon of the peroneus longus muscle, still superficial to the extensor digitorum longus. This nerve divides into two sensory branches proximal to the extensor retinaculum of the dorsal foot. Both branches run superficial to the extensor retinaculum; they are called the *medial and intermediate, dorsal cutaneous nerves of the foot.*

6.2 Motor Innervation and Testing

6.2.1 Buttock/Thigh Group

Immediately after exiting the pelvis, the sciatic nerve provides two common motor branches to innervate the hamstring muscles (▶ Fig. 6.5). One branch originates from the tibial division; the other from the common peroneal division. These hamstring branches pass distally with the sciatic nerve in the buttock region. The sciatic nerve also gives supplementary branches to the hamstring muscles as it passes next to them in the more distal thigh; however, loss of these smaller branches, in general, may not be noticed clinically when the larger, proximal hamstring branches are preserved. Considering the origin of the main hamstring branches near the pelvis, an isolated sciatic nerve injury involving the hamstring muscles would have to be very proximal (e.g., the buttock region).

The tibial portion of the sciatic nerve innervates the medial hamstrings (the *semitendinous* and *semimembranous),* as well as the *long head of the biceps femoris.* The *short head of the biceps femoris* is the only hamstring innervated by the more lateral common peroneal division of the sciatic nerve. The hamstrings (L5–S2) are tested with the patient seated and instructed to flex the knee against resistance. The examiner should simultaneously palpate the hamstring tendons in the proximal popliteal fossa (▶ Fig. 6.6). The hamstrings may also be tested with the patient prone. An isolated lesion affecting only the tibial half of the sciatic nerve spares the peroneal-innervated short head of the biceps femoris.

The tibial portion of the sciatic nerve also innervates the ischial half of the *adductor magnus* (L4 of L2–L4). Test this muscle, along with the other hip adductors (innervated by the obturator nerve), by having the patient bring the knees together against resistance, either seated (▶ Fig. 6.7) or supine.

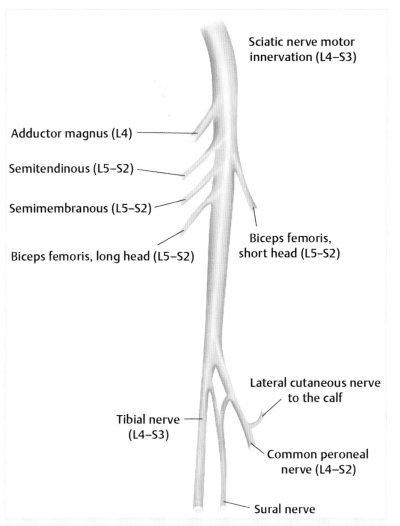

Sciatic nerve motor
innervation (L4–S3)

Adductor magnus (L4)

Semitendinous (L5–S2)

Semimembranous (L5–S2)

Biceps femoris, long head (L5–S2)

Biceps femoris,
short head (L5–S2)

Lateral cutaneous nerve
to the calf

Tibial nerve
(L4–S3)

Common peroneal
nerve (L4–S2)

Sural nerve

Fig. 6.5 Motor innervation from the sciatic (schematic) nerve in the buttock and thigh.

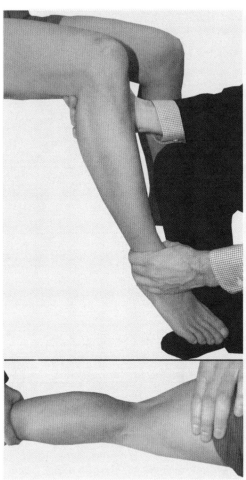

Fig. 6.6 Hamstring (L5–S2) assessment: The hamstrings are tested with the patient seated. Instruct the patient to flex the knee against resistance. The examiner should palpate the hamstring tendons in the proximal popliteal fossa. The hamstrings may also be tested with the patient prone (lower image).

6.2.2 Lower Leg

Tibial Nerve Group

The tibial nerve innervates the posterior compartment muscles of the lower leg, which control plantar flexion, foot inversion, and toe flexion (▶ Fig. 6.8). Prior to passing deep to the *gastrocnemius* and *soleus* (S1, S2), the tibial nerve sends branches to innervate these muscles. Therefore, damage to the tibial nerve deep to these muscles would spare their innervation. Although both

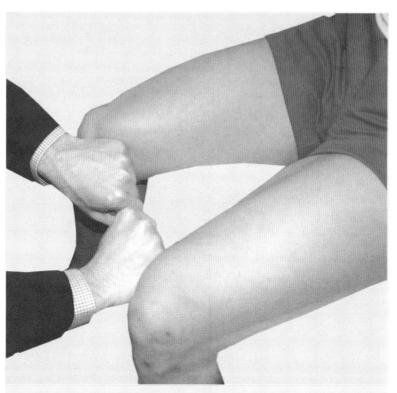

Fig. 6.7 Hip adduction (L2–L4) assessment: Test hip adduction by having the patient bring the knees together against resistance, with the patient either seated or supine. (The sciatic nerve provides only L4 contribution; L2 and L3 contribution is carried by the obturator nerve.)

the gastrocnemius (medial and lateral heads) and soleus muscles insert into the calcaneus, they have different origins. The gastrocnemius originates from the distal femur and therefore produces plantar flexion with the knee straight. In contrast, the soleus originates from the tibia and therefore can mediate plantar flexion with the knee straight or bent. Because the gastrocnemius is so powerful with the knee straight, soleus-mediated plantar flexion is only dominant when the knee is flexed. With the patient sitting, the gastrocnemius heads can be tested by extending the knee and having the patient plantar flex the foot against resistance ("pushing down on the gas pedal") (▶ Fig. 6.9). Gastrocnemius contraction can be palpated. The soleus is tested in near-isolation by instructing the patient to go up on the toes while seated with

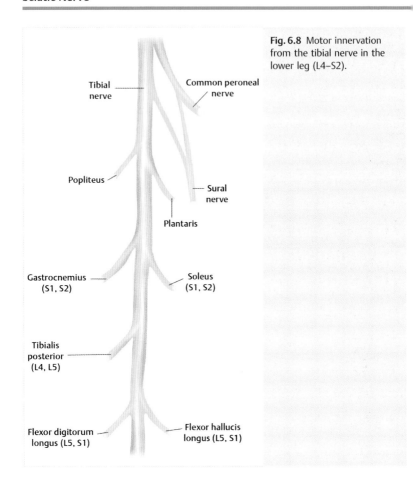

Fig. 6.8 Motor innervation from the tibial nerve in the lower leg (L4–S2).

the knee flexed (▶ Fig. 6.10). To observe subtle plantar flexion weakness, the patient should attempt to stand on the toes, one foot at a time.

Immediately deep to the soleus, the tibial nerve innervates the *tibialis posterior* (L4, L5). This muscle is the prime inverter of the foot, with its tendon inserting into the tarsal bones on the medial aspect of the foot, as well as on the lateral aspect after passing underneath the foot. Test the tibialis posterior by having the patient invert the foot against resistance (▶ Fig. 6.11). Toe flexors should remain relaxed to avoid muscular substitution. Alternatively, the patient can place the soles of the feet together while in a sitting position.

In the posterior leg compartment, the tibial nerve also innervates the *flexor digitorum longus* and the *flexor hallucis longus* (L5, S1). Tendons from these

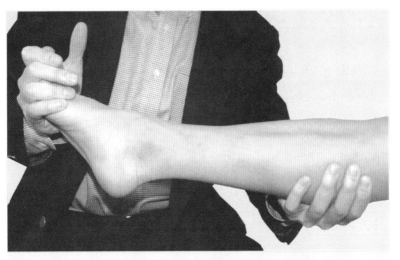

Fig. 6.9 Gastrocnemius (S1, S2) assessment: With the patient sitting, the gastrocnemius heads are tested by having the patient plantar flex the ankle against resistance with the knee straight. The examiner's other hand stabilizes the leg and palpates gastrocnemius contraction. To observe subtle plantar flexion weakness, the patient should attempt to stand on the toes, one foot at a time, or even walk on the toes.

muscles insert into the most distal phalanges of the toes, and thereby mediate flexion in all the joints they cross. To assess these muscles (along with the similar-acting flexor digitorum brevis), one instructs the patient to curl the toes against resistance. Resistance is applied by grasping the foot with both hands, using the fingers to hold the dorsum of the foot while both thumbs force the toes back into extension (▶ Fig. 6.12). The flexor hallucis longus acts on the great toe, whereas the flexor digitorum longus inserts into the rest.

♦ Together, the long toe flexors, peroneus muscles, and tibialis posterior can substitute for plantar flexion. This substitution, however, mostly flexes the forefoot, not necessarily the ankle.
♦ In the distal popliteal fossa, the tibial nerve innervates the *popliteus* and *plantaris* muscles. These two muscles have minimal clinical significance.

Deep Peroneal Nerve Group

The deep peroneal nerve innervates most of the anterior lower leg muscles, excluding the peroneus longus and brevis, which are innervated by the superficial peroneal nerve (▶ Fig. 6.13). Immediately after passing deep to the extensor digitorum longus, the deep peroneal nerve gives a motor branch to the

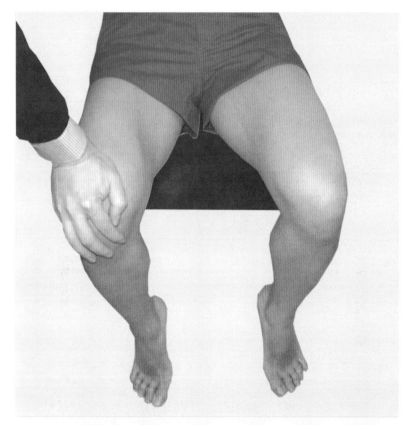

Fig. 6.10 Soleus (S1, S2) assessment: The soleus is tested in near-isolation by instructing the patient to go up on the toes while seated, with resistance placed on top of the knees.

tibialis anterior (L4–S1), which is the prime dorsiflexor of the foot. Weakness of the tibialis anterior, with sparing of the peroneus muscles, indicates an injury to the deep peroneal nerve near its origin at the fibula. Contraction of the tibialis anterior can be seen and palpated during muscle testing (▶ Fig. 6.14). The toes should remain relaxed, because contraction of the toe extensors can substitute for foot dorsiflexion.

The deep peroneal nerve innervates the *extensor digitorum longus* (L5, S1) and *extensor hallucis longus* (L5). Tendons from these muscles insert into the distal phalanges and are tested by having the patient extend the toes against resistance (▶ Fig. 6.15 and ▶ Fig. 6.16). Upon contraction, the extensor hallucis longus tendon should readily bowstring proximal to the great toe.

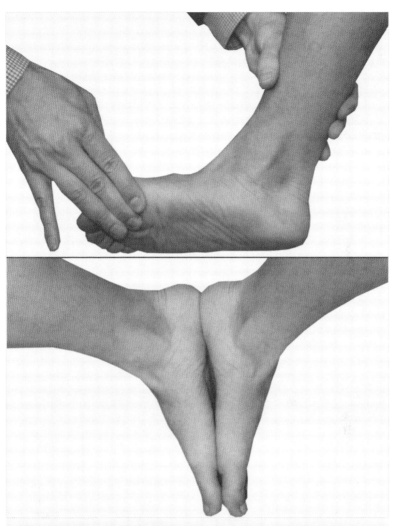

Fig. 6.11 Tibialis posterior (L4, L5) assessment: The patient inverts the foot against resistance, which tests the tibialis posterior. Toe flexors should remain relaxed to avoid substitution. Alternatively, the patient can place the soles of the feet together while in a sitting position (lower image).

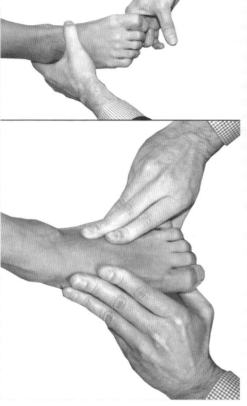

Fig. 6.12 Flexor digitorum longus, flexor hallucis longus (both L5, S1), and flexor digitorum brevis (S1, S2) assessment: To assess toe flexion, instruct the patient to curl the toes against resistance. Alternatively, resistance can be applied by grasping the foot with both hands, using the fingers to hold the dorsum of the foot while both thumbs force the toes back into extension (lower image).

♦ The motor branch destined for the extensor hallucis longus passes for a significant distance adjacent to the fibular shaft and therefore may be selectively injured with fractures or surgical procedures in this area.

6.2.3 Superficial Peroneal Nerve Group

The superficial peroneal nerve mediates foot eversion by innervating the *peroneus longus* and *brevis* (L5, S1) in the anterolateral aspect of the lower leg (▶ Fig. 6.17). These muscles originate from the fibula and insert into the foot after passing around the posterior aspect of the lateral malleolus. The peroneus brevis simply inserts into the undersurface of the fifth metatarsal. The pero-

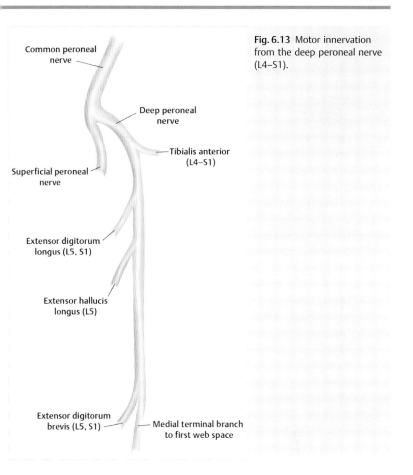

Fig. 6.13 Motor innervation from the deep peroneal nerve (L4–S1).

Common peroneal nerve

Deep peroneal nerve

Tibialis anterior (L4–S1)

Superficial peroneal nerve

Extensor digitorum longus (L5, S1)

Extensor hallucis longus (L5)

Extensor digitorum brevis (L5, S1)

Medial terminal branch to first web space

neus longus, however, mirroring the tibialis posterior, loops around the undersurface of the foot to insert into the proximal portion of the first metatarsal. The peroneus muscles are evaluated by having the patient evert the foot against resistance (▶ Fig. 6.18). Contraction of these muscles can be observed and palpated. The peroneus brevis tendon bowstrings the skin between the lateral malleolus and its insertion into the fifth metatarsal head.

♦ Although not present in most people, a lateral extension of the extensor digitorum longus, called the *peroneus tertius,* may be present. This muscle is innervated by the *superficial* peroneal nerve (not the deep peroneal nerve that innervates the extensor digitorum longus), and inserts into the fifth metatarsal. It mediates "extension" of the foot's lateral aspect.

155

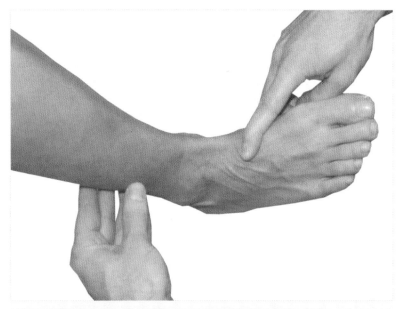

Fig. 6.14 Tibialis anterior (L4–S1) assessment: Contraction of this muscle can be seen during foot dorsiflexion. The toes should remain relaxed because the toe extensors may substitute for foot dorsiflexion.

6.2.4 Foot

Medial Plantar Nerve Group

While passing between the *abductor hallucis* and *flexor digitorum brevis* (S1, S2), the medial plantar nerve innervates these muscles (▶ Fig. 6.19). The tendons of the flexor digitorum brevis insert into the proximal phalanges of the second through fifth toes and mediate flexion at the metatarsal–phalangeal joints. More distally, the medial plantar nerve innervates the *flexor hallucis brevis* (S1, S2), which flexes the metatarsal–phalangeal joint of the great toe. These small foot muscles are difficult to isolate on examination; however, composite toe flexion can be tested (▶ Fig. 6.20). When the patient curls the arch of the foot medially, the abductor hallucis usually contracts well enough to be tested. When denervated, atrophy of the abductor hallucis may be seen. In contrast, wasting of the flexor digitorum brevis is usually not noticeable because of the thick sole and plantar aponeurosis overlying it. The medial plantar nerve usually innervates the *first lumbrical* (L5, S1) of the foot.

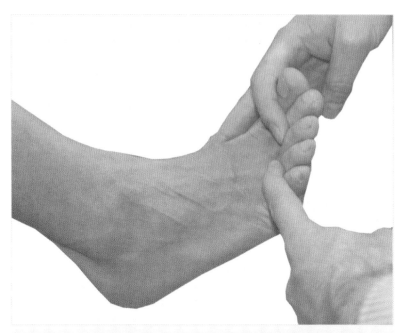

Fig. 6.15 Extensor digitorum longus (L5, S1) assessment: Have the patient extend the toes, with or without resistance.

Lateral Plantar Nerve Group

The lateral plantar nerve and its deep branch innervate most of the intrinsic muscles of the foot, analogous to the ulnar nerve in the hand (see ▶ Fig. 6.19). These muscles include the *quadratus plantae, abductor digiti minimi pedis, second to fourth lumbricals,* all the *dorsal interossei,* and both heads of the *adductor hallucis* (all via S1–S3). Foot intrinsic muscles innervated by other nerves include the abductor hallucis, flexor digitorum brevis, and flexor hallucis brevis (medial plantar nerve), as well as two muscles on the dorsum of the foot, the extensors digitorum and hallucis brevis (deep peroneal nerve, discussion follows). One may grossly assess intrinsic motor function by instructing the patient to "cup" the foot (see ▶ Fig. 6.20). Action of the individual foot intrinsic muscles cannot be readily isolated on physical examination. Chronic, severe intrinsic foot muscle weakness can cause clawing of the toes.

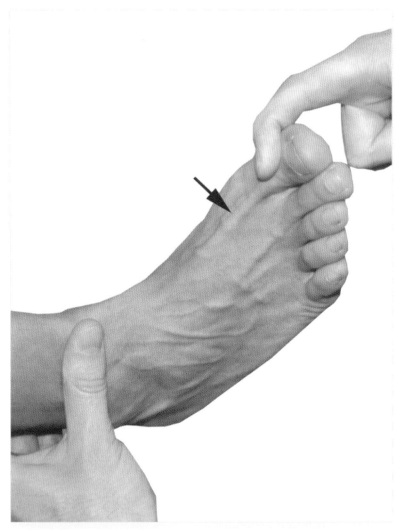

Fig. 6.16 Extensor hallucis longus (L5) assessment: Have the patient extend the great toe against resistance. The tendon (arrow) should readily bowstring proximal to the great toe.

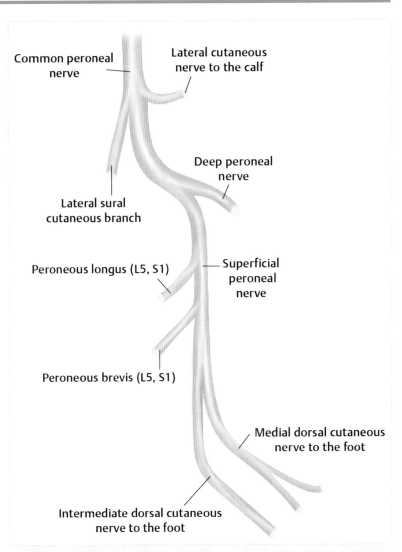

Common peroneal
nerve

Lateral cutaneous
nerve to the calf

Deep peroneal
nerve

Lateral sural
cutaneous branch

Peroneous longus (L5, S1)

Superficial
peroneal
nerve

Peroneous brevis (L5, S1)

Medial dorsal cutaneous
nerve to the foot

Intermediate dorsal cutaneous
nerve to the foot

Fig. 6.17 Motor innervation of the superficial peroneal nerve (L5–S1).

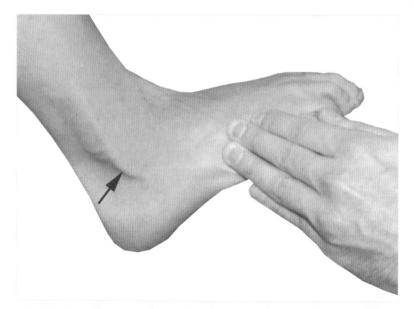

Fig. 6.18 Peroneus longus and brevis (L5, S1) assessment: The peroneus muscles are evaluated by having the patient evert the foot against resistance. Contraction of these muscles can be observed and palpated. The tendon (arrow) of the peroneus brevis can be observed bowstringing the skin between the lateral malleolus and its insertion into the fifth metatarsal head.

Deep Peroneal Nerve Group

The lateral terminal branch of the deep peroneal nerve in the dorsum of the foot innervates the *extensor digitorum brevis* (L5, S1). This muscle extends the toes at the metatarsal–phalangeal joint, a movement that is difficult to isolate from the extensors digitorum and hallucis longus. The best way to determine paralysis of the extensor digitorum brevis is to observe and palpate its contraction during composite toe extension (▶ Fig. 6.21).

6.3 Accessory Peroneal Nerve

The accessory peroneal nerve is a distal branch of the superficial peroneal nerve that is present in approximately 20% of people. When present, this branch carries motor innervation to the extensor digitorum brevis, a muscle that is usually controlled by the deep peroneal nerve. When evaluating electrophysiological and clinical examination results, one should keep this variation in mind when localizing a lesion.

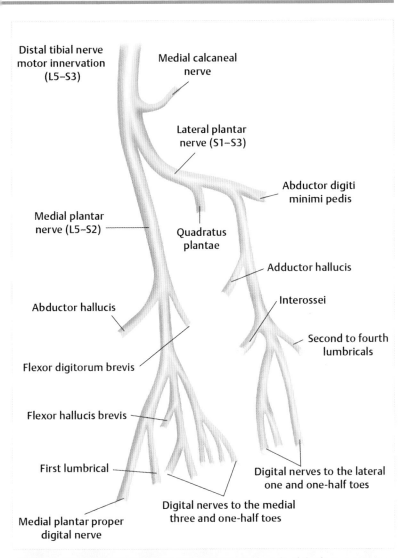

Distal tibial nerve
motor innervation
(L5–S3)

Medial calcaneal
nerve

Lateral plantar
nerve (S1–S3)

Abductor digiti
minimi pedis

Medial plantar
nerve (L5–S2)

Quadratus
plantae

Adductor hallucis

Interossei

Abductor hallucis

Second to fourth
lumbricals

Flexor digitorum brevis

Flexor hallucis brevis

First lumbrical

Digital nerves to the lateral
one and one-half toes

Medial plantar proper
digital nerve

Digital nerves to the medial
three and one-half toes

Fig. 6.19 Motor innervation from the plantar nerves in the sole of the foot.

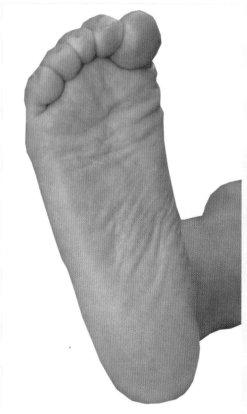

Fig. 6.20 Cupping of the sole (S1–S3): Grossly assess intrinsic motor function by instructing the patient to "cup" the foot. Alternatively, the patient can spread the toes; however, some patients with normal motor function are not able to do this. Action of the individual foot intrinsic muscles cannot be easily isolated on physical examination.

♦ The accessory peroneal nerve may occasionally originate from the deep peroneal nerve.

6.4 Sensory Innervation

The *sural nerve* provides sensory coverage to the lower lateral leg, some lateral heel and ankle, and the dorsolateral aspect of the foot, especially its lateral margin (▶ Fig. 6.22). Because of overlap in sensory coverage of the lower leg and foot, damage to the sural nerve (e.g., following an excisional biopsy) usually manifests only as numbness along the lateral border of the foot. With time, however, this area of numbness shrinks as the neighboring sensory nerves branch to partially cover the loss. The sural nerve is created by two

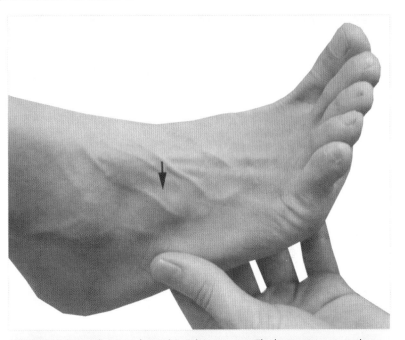

Fig. 6.21 Extensor digitorum brevis (L5, S1) assessment: The best way to assess the extensor digitorum brevis is to observe and palpate its contraction during toe extension (arrow).

communicating branches, one from the tibial nerve and the other from the common peroneal nerve. The tibial nerve gives the medial sural cutaneous nerve in the popliteal fossa whose distal continuation becomes the sural nerve proper. The common peroneal nerve in the popliteal fossa yields two sensory branches, the lateral sural cutaneous and the lateral cutaneous nerve to the calf. The first of which, as the name implies, carries fibers destined for the sural nerve. The medial and lateral sural cutaneous nerves merge just distal to the two heads of the gastrocnemius muscle.

The *lateral cutaneous nerve to the calf* provides sensory coverage of the lateral knee and calf (i.e., the upper lateral aspect of the lower leg). The remaining lower lateral portion of the leg is covered by the sural nerve, the lateral sural cutaneous branch, or cutaneous branches off the superficial peroneal nerve. The lateral cutaneous nerve to the calf does not have a consistent autonomous region to test.

Together, the deep and superficial peroneal nerves provide sensation to the dorsum of the foot and anterolateral shin (▶ Fig. 6.23). The *superficial peroneal*

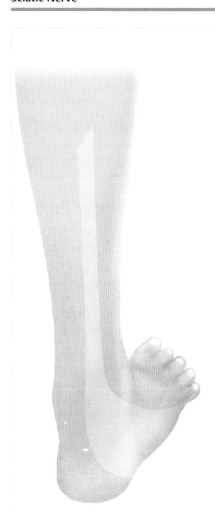

Fig. 6.22 The sural nerve. This nerve provides sensory coverage to the lower lateral leg, some lateral heel and ankle, and the dorsolateral aspect of the foot, especially its lateral margin. Because of the overlap of sensory coverage in the leg and foot, sural nerve damage (e.g., following an excisional biopsy) usually manifests only as numbness along the lateral border of the foot.

Sural nerve
sensory territory

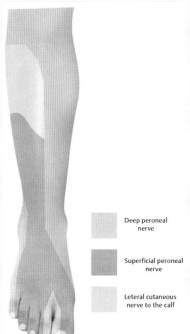

Fig. 6.23 Peroneal division sensory territory. Together, the deep and superficial peroneal nerves provide sensation to the dorsum of the foot and anterolateral shin. The superficial peroneal nerve carries the majority of this sensation, except for a small area of skin centered on the web space between the first and second toes, which the deep peroneal nerve carries. The lateral cutaneous nerve to the calf is a branch of the common peroneal nerve prior to its bifurcation.

Deep peroneal
nerve

Superficial peroneal
nerve

Leteral cutaneous
nerve to the calf

nerve carries the majority of this sensation, except for a small area of skin centered on the web space between the first and second toes covered by the *deep peroneal nerve.*

The tibial division of the sciatic nerve carries the most important sensation of the lower extremity—that for the sole of the foot (▶ Fig. 6.24). With numbness in the sole of the foot, minor trauma, or unrecognized, persistent pressure, may cause ulcers, and infection, and can even lead to amputation. Furthermore, dysesthesias in this region may prevent ambulation and be very problematic. The tibial nerve's coverage of the foot's plantar aspect is divided into three zones. The *medial calcaneal nerve* exits the tibial nerve just prior to, or within, the tarsal tunnel, and innervates the medial half of the heel. The *medial* and *lateral plantar nerves* provide sensory branches to the medial and lateral sole, respectively. The medial plantar nerve covers more area, including the first three and a half toes. The lateral plantar nerve covers the lateral one and a half toes. The plantar nerve's sensory coverage includes the nails and skin surrounding the nails on the toes' dorsal surfaces. A variable branch of the sural nerve covers sensation on the lateral heel.

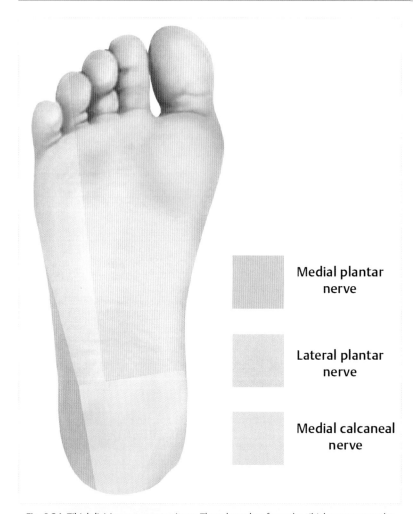

Fig. 6.24 Tibial division sensory territory. Three branches from the tibial nerve cover the foot's plantar aspect. The medial calcaneal nerve exits the tibial nerve just prior, or within, the tarsal tunnel, and innervates the medial half of the heel. The medial and lateral plantar nerves provide sensory branches to the medial and lateral sole, respectively.

6.5 Clinical Findings and Syndromes

6.5.1 Buttock

Trauma, Fractures, and Injections

A complete sciatic nerve lesion is a severe deficit. Sensation to the lateral aspect of the leg and nearly all of the foot is lost. The only sensation remaining in the foot is near the medial malleolus, which is carried by the saphenous nerve. This sensory loss is probably the most dangerous aspect of a sciatic nerve palsy—it may lead to amputation. Proper shoes and daily foot checks by the patient are mandatory until sensation returns in the sole and foot. Regarding motor control, all foot and ankle movements are lost, which in itself precludes useful ambulation without an orthotic. Loss of knee flexion can also occur for complete, proximal sciatic nerve palsies. Hamstring weakness, however, is uncommon because the major branches to these muscles originate from the sciatic nerve quite proximally, sometimes at or within the sciatic notch. For this reason, most sciatic nerve palsies actually spare knee flexion.

Care must be taken when attempting to differentiate sciatic nerve palsy from a sacral plexus injury. Making this differentiation is often not possible using just the neurological examination. With sacral plexus lesions, the gluteal nerves, pudendal nerve, and posterior cutaneous nerve to the thigh may be affected. However, a sciatic notch injury may simultaneously involve all of these nerves, along with the sciatic nerve, where they exit the pelvis. The pudendal nerve is the farthest away from the sciatic nerve in the buttock; therefore, a deficit in this nerve may be the strongest evidence on examination of a sacral lesion. For sacral plexus injury patients, imaging and electrophysiological studies are usually required.

One common cause of a buttock-level sciatic lesion is an injection injury. The safest way to administer a buttock injection is to have the patient lie prone, and then place the injection in the upper outer quadrant. Standing bent over a sink or table, or rolling over in bed is not acceptable because the topographical anatomy of the buttock becomes distorted, especially in the elderly, who have reduced amounts of subcutaneous adipose tissue and sagging buttocks. The most dangerous injection quadrant is the superomedial one. Injection injuries are readily diagnosed, considering sciatic pain and deficits characteristically begin immediately after the offending injection. Occasionally, injection injuries can present minutes to hours after an injection; the cause of this delay is uncertain. Some believe it is irritation of the nerve by the offending substance being injected in or near the epineurium. Although sciatic nerve injection injuries can cause severe motor and sensory deficits, a mild neurological deficit with persistent sciatica is most common.

Other causes of buttock-level sciatic lesions include hip fractures and orthopedic procedures. This is because the sciatic nerve runs just dorsal to the hip joint, and is separated from it by only a few thin muscles. It is vulnerable to hematomas, adjacent hardware, intraoperative retraction or coagulation, and fracture/dislocations. Of note, when isolated hip fractures injure a peripheral nerve they usually affect only the sciatic nerve. In contrast, pelvic and sacral fractures often involve the sacral plexus. Penetrating trauma can also damage the sciatic nerve in the buttock region, despite the overlying gluteus maximus.

Piriformis Syndrome

After exiting the pelvis, the sciatic nerve passes under the pyriformis muscle, which runs from the inner lateral margin of the sacrum to the greater trochanter of the femur (see ▶ Fig. 6.1). Occasionally, the sciatic nerve runs over, or through, the pyriformis muscle. Definite confirmation that pyriformis syndrome is a true clinical entity is pending, with many experts doubting its occurrence. Some have suggested pyriformis syndrome be categorized as neurogenic (with objective clinical findings) or non-neurogenic (without objective clinical findings). Patients with pyriformis syndrome have buttock and sciatic nerve distribution pain, usually without objective weakness or sensory loss on examination. Electrodiagnostic testing is usually normal. Many of these patients are originally thought to have lumbar disk herniations; either a normal lumbar spine magnetic resonance imaging scan or failed spine surgery leads to the diagnosis of pyriformis syndrome. A steroid or botulinum toxin injection into the pyriformis muscle may help ascertain the diagnosis but is not without risk. Pyriformis syndrome patients can have a history of a short fall, landing on their buttocks. If the patient is a woman and her symptoms are cyclical, one should consider focal nerve compression near the sciatic notch from endometriosis.

6.5.2 Thigh

Complete and Partial Lesions

Injuries to the sciatic nerve in the thigh region are usually caused by gunshot wounds, and less commonly by lacerations. Femur fractures or repairs may also damage the sciatic nerve. Because the main branches to the hamstrings originate in the buttock region, even complete thigh-level sciatic lesions spare knee flexion. Although the tibial and peroneal divisions of the sciatic nerve do not split from one another until the lower third of the thigh, even upper thigh and buttock lesions may predominantly, or solely, involve just one of these divisions. This is because the tibial and peroneal divisions remain separate, even though they share a common epineurium as the sciatic nerve.

Compared with the tibial division, the peroneal division is more susceptible to injury. Peroneal division injuries are also characteristically more severe, with recovery less likely. There are at least six potential reasons for this: (1) the peroneal division lies lateral and more superficial in the buttock region, making it more susceptible to trauma; (2) it is fixed between two anatomical points, the sciatic notch and the lateral fibular head, unlike the tibial nerve, which is only fixed at the sciatic notch; (3) it has less blood supply than the tibial division; (4) it has fewer and larger fascicles with less intervening connective tissue (less tensile strength); (5) peroneal-innervated muscles (e.g., peroneus longus and brevis) are themselves often concurrently injured with leg trauma; and (6) the peroneal division innervates long, thin extensor muscles, which often require robust reinnervation prior to them functioning.

6.5.3 Knee/Lower Leg

Tibial Palsy

A tibial palsy manifests as plantar flexion (gastrocnemius, soleus), foot inversion (tibialis posterior), toe flexion (flexors digitorum and hallucis longus, flexors digitorum and hallucis brevis), and foot intrinsic muscle weakness. Sensory loss occurs in the sole of the foot and the medial heel. Depending on the tibial division's contribution to the sural nerve, this nerve's sensory territory may also be affected. The most common causes of knee/lower leg tibial nerve injury are lacerations (knee level mostly) and tibia/ankle fractures and dislocations. Branches to the gastrocnemius and soleus originate proximal to the tibial nerve's passage below these muscles. Therefore, when these muscles are weak, the lesion is in, or proximal to, the popliteal fossa. Sparing of the tibialis posterior (foot inversion) helps localize a tibial lesion to the deep posterior compartment of the lower leg. Furthermore, sparing of the flexors digitorum and hallucis longus places the lesion to the lower third of the lower leg, or even distal to the tarsal tunnel. Baker cysts or other mass lesions can also cause tibial palsies at the knee. Without a history of trauma, the examiner should thoroughly palpate the popliteal fossa for masses.

Common Peroneal Nerve Palsy

Peroneal nerve damage at the knee/lower leg is usually a stretch/contusion injury, often with a concomitant fracture (e.g., a sports injury). Damage to this nerve is not uncommon because it is superficial and fixed near the lateral fibular head. Of note, peroneal nerve palsy is the most common lower-extremity nerve injury occurring after trauma. Tibiofibular joint ganglion cysts, adjacent or even within the common peroneal nerve, may also cause a peroneal nerve deficit at the knee.

Idiopathic entrapment of the common peroneal nerve occurs below the fibrous edge of the peroneus longus muscle at the fibular head (i.e., the fibular tunnel) (▶ Fig. 6.25). Diabetics are especially prone to this problem. When entrapment occurs, both the superficial and the deep peroneal branches are involved to a variable degree. Sometimes, an isolated palsy to the deep peroneal nerve may occur when this branch passes under the fibrous edge of the extensor digitorum longus muscle. Patients with common peroneal nerve entrapment have pain and numbness in a peroneal distribution (i.e., over the dorsum of the foot), radiating down from the fibular head. The lateral cutaneous nerve of the calf is spared because it does not pass through the fibular

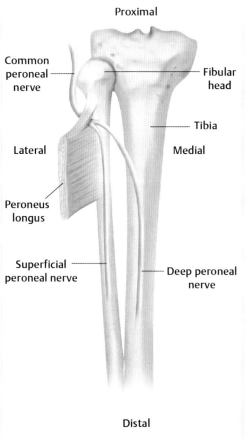

Fig. 6.25 Peroneal nerve entrapment at the fibular head. Idiopathic entrapment of the common peroneal nerve may occur at the fibular head when this nerve passes below the fibrous edge of the peroneus longus muscle. Sometimes, an isolated palsy involving the deep peroneal nerve may occur when this branch passes under the fibrous edge of the extensor digitorum longus muscle.

tunnel. Weakness of foot dorsiflexion (tibialis anterior), foot eversion (peroneus longus and brevis), and toe extension (extensor digitorum longus, extensor hallucis longus, and extensor digitorum brevis) may occur with more severe lesions. A Tinel sign is often present at the fibular head. Peroneal entrapment at the fibular head must be differentiated from an L5 radiculopathy. Because the tibialis posterior is predominantly innervated by L5 via the tibial nerve, not the common peroneal nerve, weakness affecting this muscle helps one make the correct diagnosis.

Strawberry picker's palsy occurs in persons who spend extended periods in the squatting position, which causes bilateral common peroneal nerve compression at the fibular heads. External trauma affecting the common peroneal nerve at the fibular head may occur more frequently in persons who quickly lose weight *(slimmer's paralysis)*. This may be because weight loss reduces adipose tissue that usually pads the common peroneal nerve, and furthermore, the patient now is able to cross the legs, something that was more difficult when the person was heavier. Postpartum foot drop is also a known phenomenon, having a variety of causes. These include L5 radiculopathy, pressure on the lumbosacral trunk as it passes over the bony margin of the sacroiliac joint, external compression of the common peroneal nerve or its branches by the leg holders in the lithotomy position, and, in certain developing countries, from prolonged squatting.

- Posttraumatic compartment syndrome in the lower leg may involve the anterior, posterior, and/or peroneal (lateral) compartments, producing isolated nerve palsies in the deep peroneal, tibial, and superficial peroneal branches, respectively.

6.5.4 Foot

Foot Drop

Isolated foot drop, or, more specifically, weakness in the tibialis anterior, extensor hallucis longus, and peroneus muscles, is caused by nerve injury in a variety of locations, including the L5 spinal nerve, the lumbosacral trunk, the peroneal (lateral) division of the sciatic nerve in the buttock or thigh, and the common peroneal nerve. Although a patient's history may be the most useful way to make a diagnosis, the clinical examination supplemented with electromyography can be confirmatory. For example, both L5 radicular and lumbosacral trunk lesions should cause tibialis posterior and gluteal muscle weakness. However, compared with L5 radicular lesions, patients with lumbosacral trunk damage usually do not have paraspinal muscle denervation on electromyography. Patients with peroneal division sciatic injury may have denervation of the short head of the biceps femoris, with all other hamstrings being normal.

Tarsal Tunnel Syndrome

Tarsal tunnel syndrome is an uncommon entrapment involving the medial and lateral plantar nerves where they run under the flexor retinaculum, which is a ligament that connects the medial malleolus to the calcaneus (see ▶ Fig. 6.3). Patients with this syndrome commonly have a history of regional ankle trauma; therefore, postinjury fibrosis may be causative. Other etiologies include systemic disorders (e.g., rheumatoid arthritis and diabetes mellitus). Patients with tarsal tunnel syndrome complain of sole pain, numbness, and/or paresthesias, which are worsened with walking and standing but relieved with rest and elevation. The pain is usually localized to the metatarsals. Heel pain is uncommon. Pinprick, vibratory sense, and two-point discrimination can be abnormal. Complaints of weakness are uncommon, but when present, involve

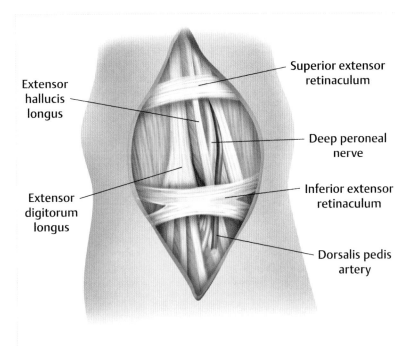

Extensor hallucis longus

Extensor digitorum longus

Superior extensor retinaculum

Deep peroneal nerve

Inferior extensor retinaculum

Dorsalis pedis artery

Fig. 6.26 Anterior tarsal tunnel anatomy (dorsal view). This syndrome is a rare cause of distal, deep peroneal nerve entrapment under one, or both, extensor retinaculums on the dorsum of the foot. Patients have dorsal foot discomfort, numbness in the first web space, and possible wasting of the extensor digitorum brevis.

he intrinsic foot muscles. A Tinel sign may be present posterior to the medial malleolus, possibly radiating down into the foot. Percussion may also cause pain radiating *up* the course of the tibial nerve, known as the *Valleix phenomenon*. Peripheral neuropathy may be differentiated from tarsal tunnel syndrome because the former usually has sensory loss outside the territory of the tibial nerve (e.g., in the sural or saphenous nerves), as well as absent ankle jerks (the ankle flexors are innervated proximal to the tarsal tunnel). Nerve conduction studies are used to help confirm the diagnosis of tarsal tunnel syndrome.

Anterior tarsal tunnel syndrome is a very rare cause of distal deep peroneal nerve entrapment under one, or both, extensor retinaculums on the dorsum of the foot (▶ Fig. 6.26). Patients have extensor digitorum brevis weakness (and/or wasting) on examination, report a dull ache on the dorsum of the foot, and sometimes have numbness localized to their first web space. A Tinel sign may occur. Tight-fitting shoes or local fibrosis following trauma may be causative.

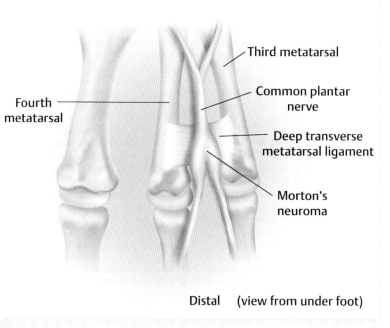

Third metatarsal

Common plantar nerve

Fourth metatarsal

Deep transverse metatarsal ligament

Morton's neuroma

Distal   (view from under foot)

Fig. 6.27 Morton's neuroma. This is actually chronic irritation of a common plantar nerve, usually the one innervating the third web space, which causes perineural fibrosis, *not* a neuroma per se. The affected nerve is pinched repetitively where it runs between the third and fourth metatarsals under the deep transverse metatarsal ligament.

Morton's Neuroma

Morton's neuroma is actually not a neuroma per se, but the chronic irritation of a common plantar nerve, usually the one innervating the third web space. This nerve usually consists of branches from both the medial and the lateral plantar nerves, and it is pinched repetitively between the third and fourth metatarsal heads where this nerve runs under the deep transverse metatarsal ligament (▶ Fig. 6.27). Intraneural fibrosis contributes to focal swelling of the nerve.

Patients with a Morton's neuroma have pain between the third and fourth metatarsals, which radiates to the third and fourth toes. The pain is worsened with walking, relieved by rest and elevation, and usually does not occur at night. Squeezing the metatarsals together can cause a shooting pain into the third and fourth toes. A Tinel sign may be present. An ultrasound examination can help make the diagnosis by documenting a swollen nerve.

7 Inguinal Complex of Nerves

7.1 Anatomical Course

A general overview of the inguinal complex of nerves' anatomical relationships with the iliopsoas muscles, pelvis, and inguinal ligament is illustrated in ▶ Fig. 7.1.

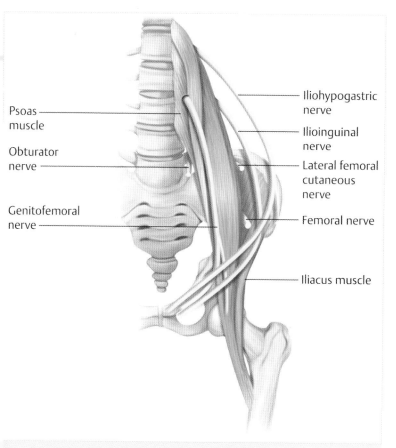

Fig. 7.1 General anatomical relationships between the inguinal complex of nerves and the psoas major, iliacus, pelvic rim, abdominal wall, and inguinal ligament.

7.1.1 Femoral Nerve

The femoral nerve is the largest branch of the lumbar plexus, being composed of the posterior divisions of the L2, L3, and L4 ventral rami (The anterior divisions of these same ventral rami make up the obturator nerve [see later discussion]). These divisional contributions to the femoral nerve merge posterior to the psoas major muscle but anterior to the transverse processes of the spine. Once formed, the femoral nerve runs inferiorly and laterally, in an oblique course down the pelvis, remaining under but near the lateral margin of the psoas major. The femoral nerve emerges from under the psoas major at the groove this muscle forms with the iliacus in the pelvis, approximately 4 cm proximal to the inguinal ligament. When the femoral nerve exits from under the psoas and passes over the iliacus muscle, it remains below the rigid iliacus fascia, which forms the roof of the *iliacus compartment.*

The femoral nerve passes deep to the inguinal ligament to enter the femoral triangle of the anterior thigh, where it remains lateral to the femoral artery (▶ Fig. 7.2). The femoral triangle is bordered by the inguinal ligament superiorly, the sartorius muscle laterally and inferiorly, and the adductor longus muscle medially. As mentioned, the femoral nerve lies deep to the iliacus fascia, which extends from the pelvis to cover and protect the femoral triangle. Of note, a small window in the iliacus fascia is present over the femoral vein and medial half of the femoral artery, just below the inguinal ligament.

A few centimeters distal to the inguinal ligament, under the sartorius muscle, the femoral nerve almost immediately splits into numerous terminal branches. These branches include three cutaneous sensory branches: the medial femoral cutaneous, intermediate femoral cutaneous, and saphenous nerves. The remaining branches are motor nerves to the quadriceps, sartorius, and pectineus. The quadriceps is composed of four muscles: the rectus femoris, vastus lateralis, vastus intermedialis, and vastus medialis. A common branch to the rectus femoris and vastus lateralis usually originates very proximal, and runs with the lateral femoral circumflex artery.

The saphenous nerve passes distal in a gradual, oblique course, from the femoral nerve near the inguinal ligament to the medial knee. The saphenous nerve runs with the femoral artery and vein, deep and parallel to the sartorius muscle, along a groove between the adductor longus and vastus medialis (subsartorial canal). The saphenous nerve then enters the adductor canal (of Hunter) with the femoral vessels, but instead of passing into the posterior compartment of the leg with them, the saphenous nerve remains anteromedial to the knee. The saphenous nerve pierces the subcutaneous fascia at, or just distal to, the knee. It provides sensory coverage to the medial leg, medial malleolus, and arch of the foot.

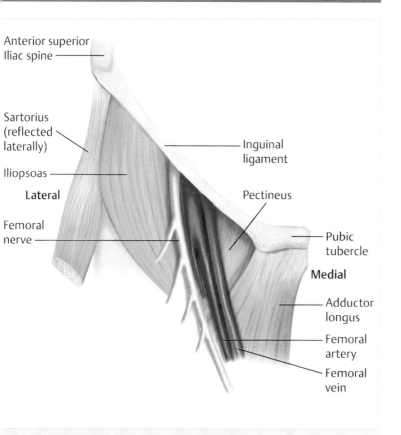

Fig. 7.2 Femoral nerve in the femoral triangle. The femoral nerve passes deep to the inguinal ligament and enters the femoral triangle of the anterior thigh, where it remains lateral to the femoral artery.

.1.2 Obturator Nerve

he obturator nerve is the second major nerve from the lumbar plexus, arising om the anterior divisions of the L2, L3, and L4 ventral rami. These spinal erve contributions fuse to form the obturator nerve in the substance of the soas major. Once formed, the obturator nerve makes its way under the psoas najor to this muscle's inferomedial border, and from there runs between the soas and the iliac vessels through the pelvis toward the obturator foramen ► Fig. 7.1). The large obturator foramen is mostly covered by the obturator

177

membrane, upon which the obturator externus muscle originates. A hole in the obturator membrane near the most superolateral aspect of the foramen is called the *obturator canal.* The obturator nerve exits the pelvis via the obturator canal (▶ Fig. 7.3).

Just prior to exiting the pelvis, the obturator nerve bifurcates into an anterior (superficial) and posterior division. Both divisions pass through the obturator

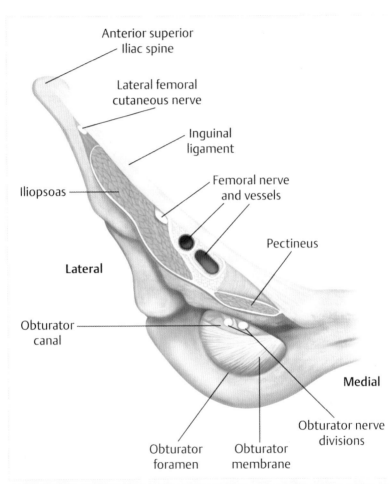

Fig. 7.3 Cross-sectional view of the inguinal region from an anterior/inferior perspective. Structures that run from the pelvis to the thigh under the inguinal ligament are depicted. The obturator nerve's divisions are shown passing through the obturator canal.

canal and perforate the obturator externus muscle, which runs from the obturator membrane to the proximal femur. Once piercing this muscle, they run deep to the pectineus muscle. The smaller, and deeper, posterior division branches upon the obturator externus, sending some branches under the adductor brevis to innervate a portion of the adductor magnus, a muscle that is also innervated by the tibial division of the sciatic nerve. The more superficial, anterior division runs over the adductor brevis, upon which it ramifies. The anterior division passes deep to the adductor longus.

A cutaneous sensory branch from the anterior division originates quite proximally, usually where this division ramifies on the adductor brevis. This cutaneous branch passes deep to the adductor longus with an oblique trajectory toward the medial, inner thigh.

➡ **A third of the population has an *accessory obturator nerve,* which originates from the anterior divisions of the L3 and L4 ventral rami. These patients have a normal, albeit smaller than usual, obturator nerve that follows its standard anatomical course. The accessory obturator nerve forms in the substance of the psoas major and passes with the normal obturator nerve medial to the psoas toward the obturator foramen. However, the accessory obturator nerve does not pass through the obturator canal, but instead passes over the superior pubic ramus. Once over the ramus, this nerve dives below the pectineus muscle to anastomose with the anterior division of the obturator nerve. When present, the accessory obturator nerve innervates the pectineus muscle, which usually receives its innervation from the femoral nerve.**

7.1.3 Lateral Femoral Cutaneous Nerve

The lateral femoral cutaneous nerve originates from the posterior divisions of the L2 and L3 ventral rami, just prior to where they join the posterior division of L4 to form the femoral nerve. The lateral femoral cutaneous nerve exits from under the psoas major, looping around and on the superior portion of the iliacus muscle toward the anterosuperior iliac crest. It then exits the pelvis just medial to the anterosuperior iliac crest, underneath the most lateral portion of the inguinal ligament. The lateral femoral cutaneous nerve usually passes under the inguinal ligament approximately 2 cm medial to the anterosuperior iliac spine.

Once outside the pelvis, it immediately splits into two or more branches, pierces the fascia, and then runs subcutaneous over the lateral aspect of the thigh. The lateral femoral cutaneous nerve and its branches usually run superficial to the sartorius muscle.

➡ **The course of the lateral femoral cutaneous nerve in the region of the anterosuperior iliac spine is variable. The nerve can pass over the iliac crest, over the inguinal ligament, or even through a small hiatus in the**

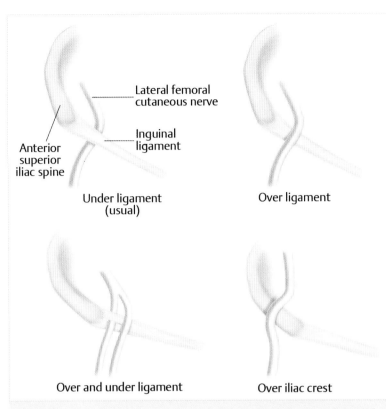

Lateral femoral
cutaneous nerve

Inguinal
ligament

Anterior
superior
iliac spine

Under ligament
(usual)

Over ligament

Over and under ligament

Over iliac crest

Fig. 7.4 Lateral femoral cutaneous nerve at the anterosuperior iliac spine. The lateral femoral cutaneous nerve usually exits the pelvis just medial to the anterosuperior iliac crest, underneath the most lateral portion of the inguinal ligament. In this region, variations in its course are the rule, with the more common ones illustrated.

ligament itself (▶ Fig. 7.4). These variations are thought to predispose an individual to idiopathic entrapment of this nerve near the iliac crest (meralgia paresthetica). It may also run under or through the sartorius muscle.

◆ The lateral femoral cutaneous nerve may originate, in part, from the femoral or genitofemoral nerves.

7.1.4 Other Nerves of the Inguinal Region

The ventral rami of T12 and L1 form a common trunk under the psoas major. This trunk then splits into the *iliohypogastric* and *ilioinguinal nerves,* with the iliohypogastric being the more superior of the two. These nerves run mostly parallel to each other, first passing through the psoas major, and then piercing its lateral margin to run over the quadratus lumborum muscle.

The iliohypogastric nerve perforates the transversus abdominis muscle over the iliac crest and then runs around the flank between this muscle and the internal oblique. Immediately superior to the anterosuperior iliac spine, a lateral branch of the iliohypogastric nerve perforates both the internal and external oblique muscles and becomes subcutaneous in the upper lateral gluteal region. The remaining portion of the iliohypogastric nerve continues toward the midline, entering the distal inguinal canal, and passes through the superficial inguinal ring to become subcutaneous in the hypogastric/suprapubic area (▸ Fig. 7.5).

The ilioinguinal nerve also passes around the flank toward the inguinal region, just caudal to the iliohypogastric nerve. The ilioinguinal nerve, however, pierces *both* the transversus abdominis and the internal oblique muscles to run between the latter and the external oblique. This nerve gives sensory branches as it runs adjacent to the spermatic cord and cremaster muscle in the inguinal canal, eventually becoming subcutaneous with the medial branch of the iliohypogastric nerve through the superficial inguinal ring (see ▸ Fig. 7.5).

The *genitofemoral nerve* is made up of branches from the L1 and L2 spinal nerves. Once formed, this nerve passes through the psoas major muscle and perforates its anterior margin just medial to the psoas minor muscle (when present). The genitofemoral nerve then passes distally adjacent to the ureter, eventually splitting into genital and femoral branches just proximal to the inguinal ligament. The femoral branch passes under the inguinal ligament just lateral to the femoral artery, becoming subcutaneous in the femoral triangle (see ▸ Fig. 7.5). The genital branch enters the deep inguinal ring, passes through the inguinal canal within the spermatic cord, and emerges from the superficial inguinal ring to innervate a portion of the genitalia.

● **A common variation is for the ilioinguinal and iliohypogastric nerves to be derived only from the L1 spinal nerve, not T12.**

7.2 Motor Innervation and Testing

7.2.1 Femoral Nerve

The femoral nerve controls hip flexion and knee extension (▸ Fig. 7.6). The first muscle innervated by the femoral nerve is the *psoas major.* Coinnervation to this muscle also arises directly from the lumbar plexus (ventral rami). The second muscle innervated by the femoral nerve is the *iliacus,* which is in the pelvis. These two muscles, along with the psoas minor, when present, insert into the proximal femur to mediate hip flexion. These muscles, collectively called the *iliopsoas* (L2–L4), are tested together by having the patient raise the

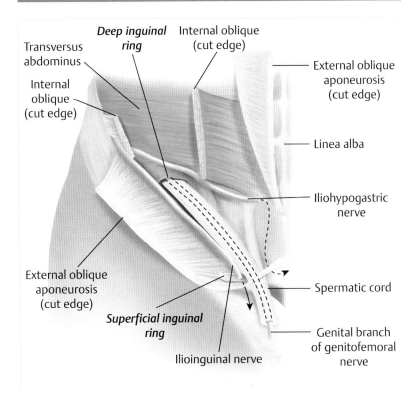

Fig. 7.5 Course of the iliohypogastric, ilioinguinal, and genitofemoral nerves in the inguinal canal (right side, anterior view). The genitofemoral nerve runs along the psoas muscle and splits into a femoral and genital branch. The femoral branch passes under the inguinal ligament, whereas the genital branch enters the deep inguinal ring to pass distally within the spermatic cord. Portions of both the iliohypogastric and the ilioinguinal nerves also pass within the inguinal canal, but not within the spermatic cord.

thigh against resistance (▶ Fig. 7.7). The patient should be either seated or supine.

Upon entering the femoral triangle and branching extensively, the femoral nerve innervates the *pectineus, sartorius,* and *quadriceps* muscles (L2–L4). The pectineus runs from the anterior pelvic rim (near the pubic tubercle) to the proximal femur. Together, the pectineus, psoas major, and iliacus form the floor of the femoral triangle, with the latter two muscles lying deeper and more lateral than the pectineus. The pectineus cannot be isolated on exam. The sarto

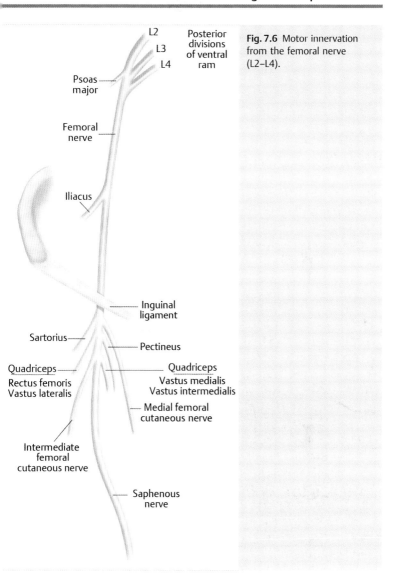

L2
L3
L4

Posterior
divisions
of ventral
ram

Fig. 7.6 Motor innervation
from the femoral nerve
(L2–L4).

Psoas
major

Femoral
nerve

Iliacus

Inguinal
ligament

Sartorius

Pectineus

Quadriceps

Rectus femoris
Vastus lateralis

Quadriceps
Vastus medialis
Vastus intermedialis

Medial femoral
cutaneous nerve

Intermediate
femoral
cutaneous nerve

Saphenous
nerve

rius, or tailor's muscle, runs from the anterosuperior iliac spine, obliquely down the leg to the medial knee, inserting into the anterior tibial tubercle. The sartorius muscle has a complex function, but in essence, abducts, flexes, and externally rotates the hip. To semi-isolate this muscle, start with the

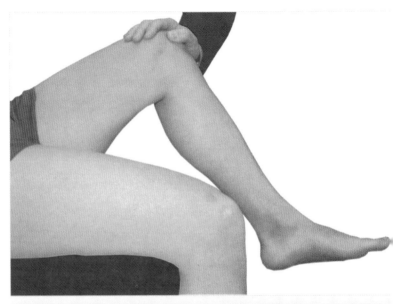

Fig. 7.7 Iliopsoas (L2–L4) assessment: The psoas major and iliacus muscles (collectively termed the iliopsoas) are tested together by having the patient raise the knee (flex the hip) against resistance, with the patient either sitting (shown) or lying supine.

patient seated. Instruct the patient to place one foot on the contralateral knee by dragging it up the shin (▶ Fig. 7.8). Contraction of the sartorius may be palpated.

The quadriceps muscles mediate lower leg extension at the knee. The *rectus femoris* and *vastus lateralis* often share a common branch from the femoral nerve; the *vastus intermedialis* and *medialis* usually have their own branches (they can also share a common branch). With the patient seated, the quadriceps are tested by applying resistance against lower leg extension (▶ Fig. 7.9). The muscle mass of the quadriceps should be observed and palpated because the sartorius (femoral nerve) and tensor fascia lata (superior gluteal nerve) may deceptively substitute for leg extension in some patients.

7.2.2 Obturator Nerve

The anterior division of the obturator nerve provides motor fibers to the *adductor brevis, adductor longus,* and *gracilis* (▶ Fig. 7.10). This pattern of muscular innervation makes sense, considering the obturator's anterior division

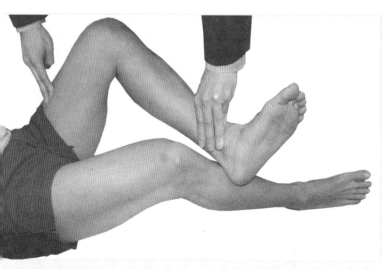

Fig. 7.8 Sartorius (L2–L4) assessment: The sartorius muscle abducts, flexes, and externally rotates the hip. To semi-isolate this muscle, start with the patient seated. Instruct the patient to place the foot on the contralateral knee by dragging it up the shin. Contraction of the sartorius may be palpated.

uns between the first two muscles and ends near the third. The posterior division innervates the *obturator externus* and terminates by innervating a small portion of the *adductor magnus,* deep to the adductor brevis. To test obturator nerve motor function (i.e., the adductors, L2–L4), have the patient squeeze the thighs together against resistance at the inner knees (▶ Fig. 7.11).

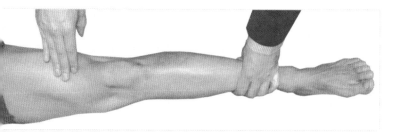

Fig. 7.9 Quadriceps (L2–L4) assessment: With the patient seated, the quadriceps are tested by applying resistance against knee extension. The quadriceps' muscle mass should be observed and palpated because the sartorius (femoral nerve) and tensor fascia lata (superior gluteal nerve) may substitute for knee extension.

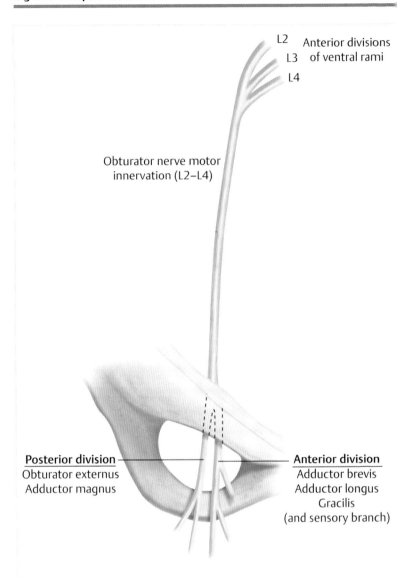

L2
L3   Anterior divisions
L4   of ventral rami

Obturator nerve motor
innervation (L2–L4)

Posterior division
Obturator externus
Adductor magnus

Anterior division
Adductor brevis
Adductor longus
Gracilis
(and sensory branch)

Fig. 7.10 Motor innervation from the obturator nerve.

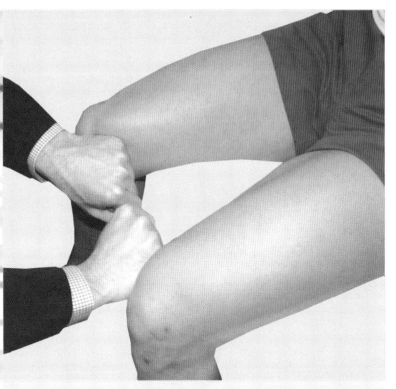

Fig. 7.11 Adductor (L2–L4) assessment: Have the patient squeeze the thighs with resistance placed at the inner knees.

♦ Innervation of the adductors is variable, with the adductors longus, brevis, and magnus often receiving innervation from either or both divisions of the obturator nerve.

7.2.3 Other Nerves of the Inguinal Region

The iliohypogastric and ilioinguinal nerves provide motor branches to the *transversus abdominis* and *internal oblique* muscles. The ilioinguinal nerve also innervates the *pyramidalis,* a muscle which, when present, can be tested with electromyography. The genital branch of the genitofemoral nerve innervates the *cremaster* muscle, which helps mediate testicular thermoregulation by elevating the ipsilateral testicle. This reflex may be tested by applying light touch to the inguinal region and observing ipsi-lateral testicular elevation.

7.3 Sensory Innervation

7.3.1 Femoral Nerve

The femoral nerve's sensory territory includes the anterior and medial thigh, as well as the medial leg and foot via the saphenous nerve (▶ Fig. 7.12). The *medial femoral cutaneous nerve* branches from the femoral nerve in the femoral triangle and carries sensation from the medial thigh, mostly distal (the proximal, medial thigh is covered more by the obturator nerve). The *intermediate femoral cutaneous nerve* also branches from the proximal femoral nerve and covers sensation on the anterior (and somewhat medial) aspect of the thigh.

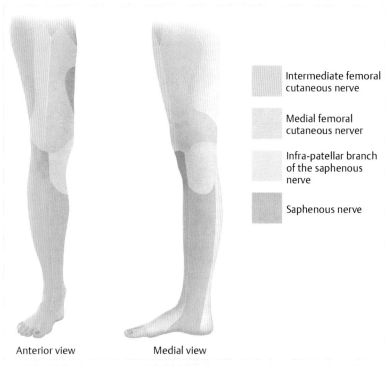

Intermediate femoral cutaneous nerve

Medial femoral cutaneous nerver

Infra-patellar branch of the saphenous nerve

Saphenous nerve

Anterior view   Medial view

Fig. 7.12 Femoral nerve sensory innervation. The femoral nerve's sensory territory includes the anterior and medial thigh, as well as the medial lower leg and foot via the saphenous nerve.

Overall, an autonomous sensory zone for the femoral nerve is over the distal, anterior thigh.

The *saphenous nerve's* sensory territory includes the medial knee, medial lower leg, medial malleolus, and arch of the foot. Mostly small, unnamed branches of the saphenous nerve provide this cutaneous innervation. On the medial knee, however, the saphenous nerve frequently has a large cutaneous branch called the *infrapatellar branch of the saphenous nerve.*

7.3.2 Obturator Nerve

As mentioned, the obturator nerve's anterior (superficial) division has a proximal sensory branch that passes under the adductor longus and perforates the subcutaneous fascia of the thigh. This branch provides sensation to the medial thigh region (▶ Fig. 7.13). Sensory loss in this area is not always present with complete obturator palsies and therefore is not considered autonomous.

7.3.3 Lateral Femoral Cutaneous Nerve

The lateral femoral cutaneous nerve's sensory territory includes the anterior, lateral aspect of the thigh (▶ Fig. 7.14). This nerve has an autonomous zone, which is located on the midlateral thigh.

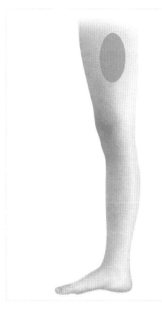

Fig. 7.13 Obturator nerve sensory innervation (medial view). The obturator nerve's anterior (superficial) division has a proximal sensory branch that passes under the adductor longus and provides sensation to the medial thigh region.

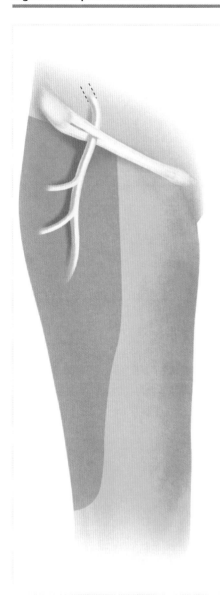

Fig. 7.14 Lateral femoral cutaneous nerve sensory innervation. This nerve's sensory territory includes the anterolateral aspect of the thigh. This nerve has an autonomous zone, which is located on the lower, lateral thigh proximal to the knee.

7.3.4 Other Nerves of the Inguinal Region

The iliohypogastric, ilioinguinal, and genitofemoral nerves all provide significant sensory coverage of the inguinal and pubic regions (▶ Fig. 7.15). Their sensory territories overlap, but semiautonomous zones do exist. The iliohypogastric nerve provides sensation to the suprapubic region. This nerve also gives a lateral cutaneous branch that passes over the iliac crest and innervates the upper, lateral buttock. The ilioinguinal nerve passes through the inguinal canal and provides sensation to the skin overlying the inguinal ligament, upper medial thigh, and mons pubis/base of the penis. For the genitofemoral nerve, its femoral branch passes under the inguinal ligament to cover the femoral triangle, whereas the genital branch passes within the spermatic cord to supply the scrotum/labia.

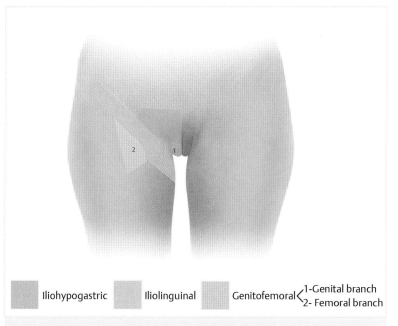

		1-Genital branch
Iliohypogastric	Iliolinguinal	Genitofemoral ⟨
		2- Femoral branch

Fig. 7.15 Sensory territory of the iliohypogastric, ilioinguinal, and genitofemoral nerves. These nerves all provide significant sensory coverage of the inguinal and pubic regions. Although their coverage overlaps, semiautonomous zones do exist. For the iliohypogastric nerve, it is the suprapubic region. For the ilioinguinal nerve, it is along the inguinal ligament. For the genitofemoral nerve, it is the femoral triangle (femoral branch) and scrotum/labia (genital branch).

7.4 Clinical Findings and Syndromes

7.4.1 Femoral Nerve

Injury to the femoral nerve is usually iatrogenic. Causes include gynecological procedures, femoral artery puncture for catheterization, arterial bypass procedures, hip surgery using methylmethacrylate, and pelvic surgery for tumors. Traditionally, an abdominal hysterectomy is the operation most frequently associated with femoral nerve damage. Trauma may also cause femoral nerve injury, including gunshot wounds to the groin and pelvis, lacerations, and hip/pelvis fractures. Expanding retroperitoneal (psoas or iliacus compartment) and femoral triangle hematomas secondary to anticoagulation, trauma, or catheter placement may also cause femoral injury. Although proximal diabetic neuropathies frequently involve the femoral nerve, this nerve is rarely affected in isolation. Usually the lumbar spinal nerves, lumbosacral plexus, and other peripheral nerves are also involved with diabetic neuropathies.

Patients with significant femoral neuropathies often complain of incoordination or buckling of the knee and not paralysis per se. These patients have trouble standing up from a seated position, as well as climbing stairs. A frontward kick is weak or impossible. Sensory loss may be confirmatory and includes the anterior thigh (intermediate femoral cutaneous nerve), lower medial thigh (medial femoral cutaneous nerve), medial knee (infrapatellar branch of the saphenous nerve), and medial lower leg and foot (saphenous nerve).

For patients with a suspected femoral neuropathy involving the iliopsoas muscle, which indicates a very proximal lesion, one should make certain to examine hip adductor strength. If hip adduction is weak, a lesion affecting the lumbar plexus, or multiple spinal nerves (i.e., L2–L4), is more likely, and imaging should be performed. Furthermore, a femoral neuropathy should be differentiated from an L4 radiculopathy. Both femoral neuropathy and L4 radiculopathy can manifest with quadriceps weakness, an absent knee jerk, and medial lower leg (shin) numbness in the saphenous territory. However, only a radiculopathy would have concurrent hip adductor (L2–L4), anterior tibialis (L4–S1), and posterior tibialis (L4–L5) weakness. Therefore, these three muscles should also be closely examined.

Idiopathic entrapment of the saphenous nerve has been reported at the adductor canal in the distal, medial thigh. Prolonged or absent sensory conduction velocities in the saphenous nerve distal to the canal may occur. Surgical release of the adductor canal may be indicated for select patients.

♦ **Rarely, patients may present with spontaneous and isolated numbness in the territory of the saphenous nerve's infrapatellar branch (i.e., *gonyalgia paresthetica*). The cause is uncertain.**

7.4.2 Obturator Nerve

Patients with obturator palsies have weak hip adduction and a variable amount of medial thigh sensory loss. The adductor tendon reflex may be absent, although this reflex may also be absent in normal subjects. Injury to the obturator nerve is rare but may be from penetrating trauma to the inguinal region or pelvis. As with the femoral nerve, iatrogenic etiologies are common and include pelvic surgery, especially for tumors. These injuries may be from direct manipulation, transection, or retractor stretch injury. Sometimes motor and sensory deficits are minimal to absent, and the patient only complains of pelvic/groin pain radiating to the medial thigh. If a neuroma occurs, then a Tinel sign may be present in the groin or lateral vaginal wall. Injury to the accessory obturator nerve may also occur where it passes over the superior pubic ramus.

To exclude a lumbar plexus lesion or radiculopathy (e.g., L3, L4) in patients with suspected obturator palsies, normal strength in the quadriceps and an active knee jerk should be documented.

Idiopathic obturator nerve entrapment by a fibrous arch in the obturator canal has been reported. These patients present with groin discomfort and pain radiating to the medial thigh. Although adductor strength is often normal in these patients, needle electromyography of the hip adductors may help confirm the diagnosis. A test infiltration of anesthetic where the nerve is most tender may be therapeutically and diagnostically useful.

7.4.3 Lateral Femoral Cutaneous Nerve

Irritation of the lateral femoral cutaneous nerve is referred to as *meralgia paresthetica* (i.e., Bernhardt-Roth syndrome). Patients report numbness, paresthesias, pain, and/or hyperesthesia on the anterolateral aspect of the thigh. The etiology of this syndrome is usually considered idiopathic; however, it can be related to a repetitive trauma or irritation. Patients may report worsened pain with standing and walking, and relief with flexion at the hip or sitting. Most symptoms are mild and self-limiting. Examination reveals sensory changes, especially hyperesthesia, on the lateral thigh. One provocative examination maneuver is to extend the hip, which places the nerve on stretch and may exacerbate the patient's symptoms. Deep palpation along the lateral inguinal ligament may also be tender. A Tinel sign is usually absent. The diagnosis may be confirmed with an injection of local anesthetic near the anterosuperior iliac spine, which should ameliorate the symptoms. However, considering the anatomical variability this nerve exhibits (see ▸ Fig. 7.4), there are many false-negatives with this test. Sensory conduction velocities may aid in the diagnosis.

An anomalous course of the lateral femoral cutaneous nerve may predispose one to neuropathy. Other predisposing conditions include obesity, ascites, and pregnancy: a protuberant abdomen is thought to distort regional anatomy and predispose one to meralgia paresthetica. Conversely, extreme weight loss is also associated with this disorder. Diabetes does not appear to be related. An autosomal dominant form of familial meralgia paresthetica has been reported.

An isolated neuropathy of the lateral femoral cutaneous nerve can be readily differentiated from a femoral or lumbar plexus lesion because the latter diagnoses cause more extensive sensory loss over the anterior/medial thigh, as well as motor weakness. The more problematic differential is that from an L2 radiculopathy, which affects the upper, lateral thigh. However, an L2 radiculopathy causes pain or numbness extending more over the anterior and medial aspect of the upper thigh than expected in meralgia paresthetica. Furthermore, an L2 radiculopathy may also cause iliopsoas weakness.

7.4.4 Inguinal Neuralgia

The iliohypogastric and ilioinguinal nerves may be disrupted or damaged secondary to transverse abdominal incisions (e.g., hysterectomies or other lower-quadrant procedures), or during inguinal hernia repairs. Damage to either nerve may cause back, inguinal, and scrotal/labial pain. To confirm the diagnosis of an iliohypogastric or ilioinguinal neuropathy, three criteria should be fulfilled: (1) history of a surgical procedure involving the abdomen or pelvis, (2) sensory changes in the suprapubic area (iliohypogastric nerve) or along the inguinal ligament (ilioinguinal nerve), and (3) relief produced by anesthetic infiltration of these nerves near the anterosuperior iliac spine. As mentioned, sensory testing in the groin helps distinguish which of these two nerves is involved.

Although rare, the genitofemoral nerve may be damaged during inguinal hernia repair or gynecological procedures. Previous appendicitis or psoas abscesses can also damage this nerve on the anterior margin of the psoas muscle. Genitofemoral neuralgia pain occurs in the inguinal region, scrotum/labia, and/or femoral triangle. Focal sensory loss over the femoral triangle helps confirm this diagnosis. A local nerve block of the iliohypogastric and ilioinguinal nerves, just medial to the anterosuperior iliac spine, would fail to alleviate symptoms that are from an irritated genitofemoral nerve, which does not pass through this region. However, a paraspinal block of the L1 and L2 spinal nerves, which blocks the genitofemoral nerve (and partially the ilioinguinal and/or iliohypogastric nerves), should relieve the pain.

If a patient with inguinal neuralgia has back pain or no history of previous inguinal or abdominal surgery, than an L1 radiculopathy should be ruled out with magnetic resonance imaging.

8 Lumbosacral Plexus

8.1 Lumbar Plexus

The lumbar plexus is created from the T12–L4 ventral rami, which inter-communicate to form the anterior and posterior divisions of the lumbar plexus in the substance of the psoas major, anterior to the transverse processes (▶ Fig. 8.1). The majority of the lumbar plexus is within the psoas major muscle. A portion of L4 and all of L5 provide indirect input to the sacral plexus via the lumbar plexus.

The terminal branches of the lumbar plexus provide motor and sensory innervation to the lower abdomen, anterior thigh, and medial thigh. Besides its communication with the sacral plexus, there are six branches from the lumbar plexus: two groups of three. The first group consists of major branches to the anterior and medial thigh, whereas the second group includes minor branches to the groin. Both groups, all six branches, constitute the inguinal complex of nerves. The anatomy and function of these branches have been described in Chapter 7.

The three major branches of the lumbar plexus are the *femoral, obturator,* and *lateral femoral cutaneous nerves,* which arise from the L2, L3, and L4 spinal nerves. Shortly after exiting their respective foramina, these spinal nerves bifurcate into anterior and posterior divisions. The anterior divisions form the obturator nerve, whereas the posterior divisions form the femoral nerve. The lateral femoral cutaneous nerve arises from the posterior divisions of L2 and L3 prior to where these divisions create the femoral nerve. The lateral femoral cutaneous nerve is the most cranial of the three major branches. It emerges from the lateral margin of the psoas major and passes along the abdominal wall to the anterosuperior iliac spine, where it exits the pelvis. The femoral nerve travels down and within the posterior aspect of the psoas major and emerges in the pelvis from between this muscle and the iliacus, approximately 4 cm proximal to the inguinal ligament. In contrast to the other lumbar plexus branches, the obturator nerve runs along the *medial* aspect of the psoas major, emerges from its medial border in the pelvis, and enters the thigh via the obturator canal.

The three minor branches of the lumbar plexus to the groin are the *iliohypogastric, ilioinguinal,* and *genitofemoral nerves.* The iliohypogastric and ilioinguinal nerves arise from a common trunk, which has contribution from T12 and L1. This trunk bifurcates within the substance of the psoas major, yielding the more superior (cranial) iliohypogastric nerve (T12, L1) and the more caudal ilioinguinal nerve (only L1), both of which perforate the lateral margin of the psoas major and loop around the abdominal wall toward the inguinal ligament. After L1 and L2 form the genitofemoral nerve, this nerve perforates the

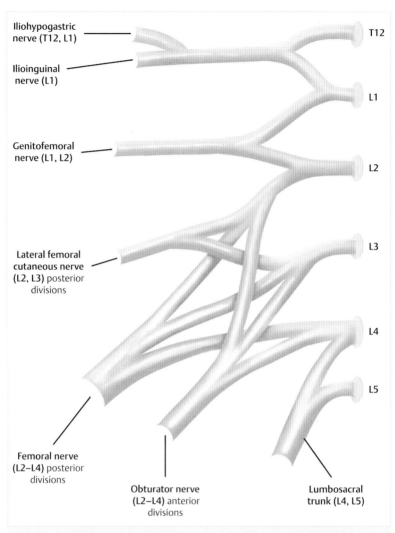

Fig. 8.1 Lumbar plexus. The lumbar plexus is composed of the T12–L4 ventral rami, which intercommunicate and coalesce to form anterior and posterior divisions in the substance of the psoas major, anterior to the transverse processes. A portion of L4, and all of L5, provides input to the sacral plexus via the lumbosacral trunk.

anterior margin of the psoas major, medial to the psoas minor, and runs caudally on this muscle next to the ureter. The ventral rami of T12–L2 (which contribute to the iliohypogastric, ilioinguinal, and genitofemoral nerves) do not divide into anterior and posterior divisions in the psoas major. This occurs only in the more caudal, major branches of the lumbar plexus already mentioned.

The lumbosacral trunk, which is composed of a portion of L4 and all of L5 (ventral rami), passes caudally over the sacral ala, adjacent to the sacroiliac joint, to join the sacral plexus. The lumbosacral trunk provides motor and sensory innervation destined for the common peroneal division of the sciatic nerve. The L4 spinal nerve is known as the *furcal nerve. Furcal* ("forked") refers to the three proximal divisions of the L4 spinal nerve (ventral ramus only): lumbosacral trunk contribution, anterior division to the obturator nerve, and posterior division to the femoral nerve.

◈ **Other small motor branches also arise directly from the lumbar plexus. For example, the ventral rami of L1 to L4 provide motor innervation to the quadratus lumborum and sometimes the psoas major. One or two proximal branches off the femoral nerve also provide motor innervation to the psoas major.**

◈ **When present, the psoas minor is innervated by small motor branches from the L1 and L2 spinal nerves.**

8.2 Sacral Plexus

The *sacral plexus* is a triangular-shaped complex of nerves that lie on the inner surface of the sacroiliac joint (▶ Fig. 8.2). It originates from the ventral rami of the L4–S4 spinal nerves; of which S1–S4 emerge from the ventral sacral foramina. The lumbosacral trunk, composed of the L4 and L5 contributions to the sacral plexus, passes medial to the obturator nerve into the lesser pelvis where it joins the sacral plexus. Similar to the lower lumbar plexus, ventral rami contributions to the sacral plexus bifurcate into anterior and posterior divisions prior to forming the plexal branches. Nearly all the anterior divisions coalesce to form the tibial division of the sciatic nerve (L4–S3). The posterior divisions, except S3 and S4, form the common peroneal division of the sciatic nerve (L4–S2). The fact that the common peroneal nerve is made of one less division makes sense, considering it is smaller than the tibial nerve.

There are several other sacral plexus branches in addition to the sciatic nerve. These branches may be categorized based on whether they originate from the anterior divisions, posterior divisions, or both.

8.2.1 Branches from the Anterior Divisions

Two branches arise from the anterior divisions of the sacral plexus. The first is the *nerve to the quadratus femoris and inferior gemelli,* which arises from the

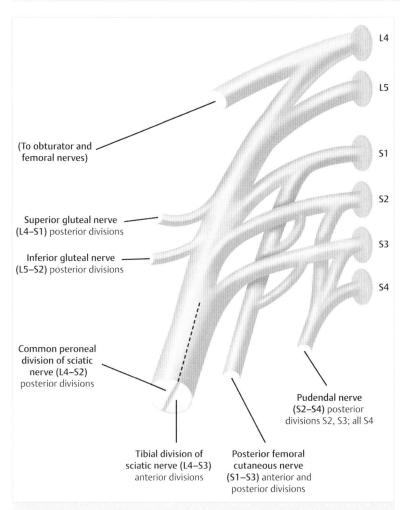

L4

L5

S1

S2

S3

S4

(To obturator and
femoral nerves)

Superior gluteal nerve
(L4–S1) posterior divisions

Inferior gluteal nerve
(L5–S2) posterior divisions

Common peroneal
division of sciatic
nerve (L4–S2)
posterior divisions

Pudendal nerve
(S2–S4) posterior
divisions S2, S3; all S4

Tibial division of
sciatic nerve (L4–S3)
anterior divisions

Posterior femoral
cutaneous nerve
(S1–S3) anterior and
posterior divisions

Fig. 8.2 Sacral plexus. The sacral plexus is a triangular complex of nerves lying on the sacroiliac joint. It is composed of ventral rami from the L4–S4 spinal nerves, of which S1–S4 emerge from the ventral sacral foramina. All spinal nerve contributions, except S4, bifurcate into anterior and posterior divisions (not shown) prior to forming terminal branches.

anterior divisions of L4, L5, and S1. The second is the *nerve to the obturator internus and superior gemelli,* which originates from the anterior divisions of L5, S1, and S2. Both of these nerves arise from three divisions; however, their origins are shifted by one spinal nerve level. They provide motor innervation to their named muscles, which together externally rotate the hip. Test this movement with the patient seated, legs dangling. While stabilizing the knee with one hand, instruct the patient to resist when you pull the lower leg inward (▶ Fig. 8.3).

8.2.2 Branches from the Posterior Divisions

There are also two branches from the posterior divisions of the sacral plexus, each similarly originating from three divisions, shifted by one spinal nerve level. The *superior gluteal nerve* arises from the posterior divisions of L4, L5, and S1, and the *inferior gluteal nerve* from the posterior divisions of L5, S1, and S2.

The superior gluteal nerve exits the pelvis through the greater sciatic foramen above the pyriformis muscle and innervates the gluteus medius, gluteus minimus, and tensor fascia latae muscles. These three muscles act in conjunction to abduct the hip. Abduction of an extended hip is from gluteus medius and minimus contraction. In contrast, abduction of a flexed hip is secondary to tensor fascia latae contraction. To test gluteus hip abduction, the patient should abduct the hip against resistance while supine or standing (▶ Fig. 8.4). Normally, you should not be able to break hip abduction. Alternatively, to test tensor fascia latae hip abduction the patient should spread the thighs while seated on an examining bench (▶ Fig. 8.5).

The inferior gluteal nerve innervates the gluteus maximus muscle, which extends the hip with some assistance from the hamstrings. The gluteus maximus may be tested in isolation with the patient either prone or standing (▶ Fig. 8.6). Start with the knee flexed to eliminate hamstring substitution and instruct the patient to extend the hip. Of note, it is normal for this range of motion to be limited, because the rectus femoris muscle is stretched when the hip is extended. The buttock may be palpated to ascertain muscle contraction.

8.2.3 Branch from the Anterior and Posterior Divisions

The *posterior femoral cutaneous nerve* originates from the anterior and posterior divisions of S1–S3. More specifically, it arises from the posterior divisions of S1 and S2, and the anterior divisions of S2 and S3. The posterior femoral cutaneous nerve is called the *lesser sciatic nerve* and runs medial and parallel to the sciatic nerve in the buttock region. As both of these "sciatic" nerves pass distally, the posterior femoral cutaneous nerve becomes more superficial and medial, running just lateral to the ischial tuberosity at the lower margin of the

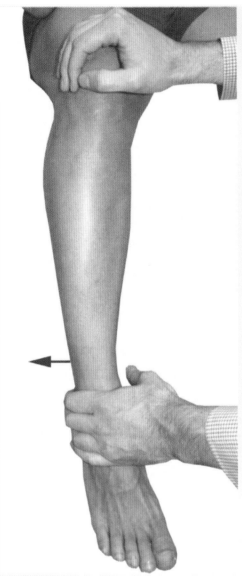

Fig. 8.3 External rotation of a flexed hip (L4–S2) assessment: Test this movement with the patient seated, legs dangling. While stabilizing the knee with one hand, instruct the patient to resist when you pull the lower leg inward.

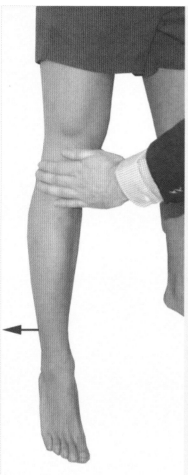

Fig. 8.4 Gluteus medius and minimus hip abduction (L4–S1) assessment: The patient should abduct an extended hip against resistance while standing (shown) or supine. Normally, you should not be able to break hip abduction.

gluteus maximus. At the gluteal fold, it pierces the fascia and becomes sub-cutaneous. Its sensory territory includes the lower buttock, posterior midline of the thigh, and most of the popliteal region (▶ Fig. 8.7). In some individuals, this territory may extend distally to include the posterior calf. Considering their close anatomical relationship, the posterior femoral cutaneous and sciatic nerves may be concurrently damaged.

Injury to the posterior femoral cutaneous nerve causes numbness in the lower buttock and posterior thigh, which may be confused with an S2 radicul-opathy. They may be differentiated because, in addition to radiating low back

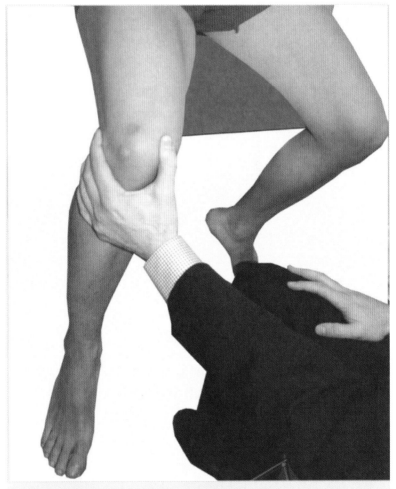

Fig. 8.5 Tensor fascia latae hip abduction (L4–S1) assessment: Have the patient spread the thighs while seated on an examining bench. By flexing the hip, contribution to hip abduction from the gluteal muscles is minimized.

pain, patients with S2 radiculopathy usually have mild gastrocnemius weakness and a depressed ankle reflex.

There are multiple branches from the posterior femoral cutaneous nerve that pierce the fascia and become subcutaneous at the gluteal fold. The more lateral branches are called the *inferior cluneal nerves* and provide sensation to

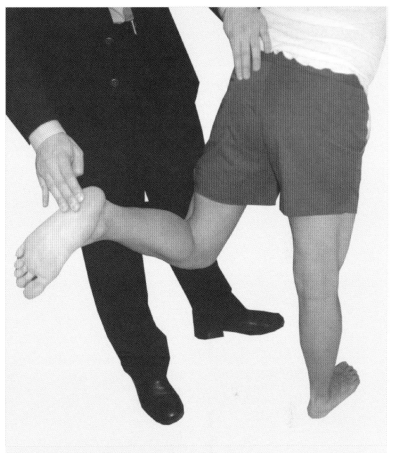

Fig. 8.6 Hip extension (L5–S2) assessment: The gluteus maximus may be tested in isolation with the patient either standing (shown) or prone. Start with the leg flexed at the knee to eliminate hamstring substitution. Instruct the patient to extend the hip. The buttock may be palpated to ascertain muscle contraction.

the inferior and lateral buttock. The large medial branch is called the *inferior pudendal nerve,* which provides sensation to the scrotum or labia.

8.2.4 Other Branches

The *pudendal nerve* primarily originates from S4, with supplemental input from the anterior divisions of both S2 and S3 spinal nerves. The pudendal

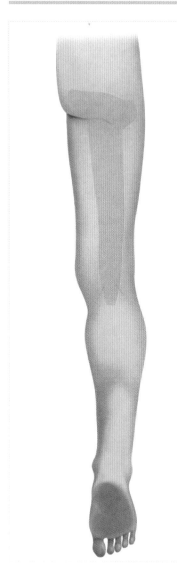

Fig. 8.7 Sensory territory of the posterior femoral cutaneous nerve (posterior view). This nerve's sensory territory includes the posterior midline of the thigh and most of the popliteal region. In some individuals, its territory may extend distally to include the posterior calf.

nerve exits the medial aspect of the greater sciatic foramen, turns to enter the lesser sciatic foramen, and makes its way to the pudendal (Alcock's) canal, which is deep to the sacrospinous ligament (▶ Fig. 8.8). There are three named branches of the pudendal nerve: (1) the inferior rectal nerve, which innervates

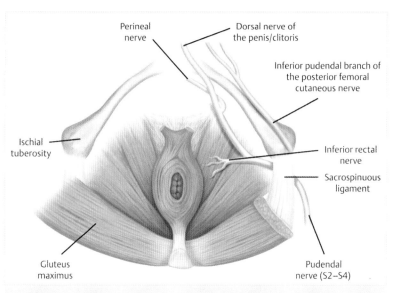

Fig. 8.8 Branches of the pudendal nerve (caudal view). The pudendal nerve exits the medial aspect of the greater sciatic foramen, turns to enter the lesser sciatic foramen, making its way through the pudendal (Alcock's) canal deep to the sacrospinous ligament. There are three pudendal nerve branches: the inferior rectal nerve, the perineal nerve (the continuation of the pudendal nerve after the inferior rectal nerve branch), and the dorsal nerve to the penis or clitoris.

the external anal sphincter and skin around the anus; (2) the perineal nerve (the continuation of the pudendal nerve after the inferior rectal nerve branch), which runs with the perineal artery to innervate the posterior scrotum or labia, erectile tissue, and external urethral sphincter; and (3) the dorsal nerve to the penis or clitoris.

Small branches from the S1 and S2 ventral rami merge to become the *nerve to the pyriformis.* The pyriformis muscle assists in external rotation of the hip when flexed (see ▶ Fig. 8.3).

♦ Similar to the brachial plexus, spinal nerve input to the lumbosacral plexus is variable. When T12 provides a large contribution, and S3 only a minimal one or none at all, the lumbosacral plexus is considered prefixed. In contrast, when T12 provides no input, L1 only a small contribution, and S4 significant input to the plexus (besides the pudendal nerve), the lumbosacral plexus is considered postfixed. Furthermore, each branch from the lumbosacral plexus may be composed of more, or less, spinal nerve components than usual.

8.3 Diagnostic Approach to the Lumbosacral Plexus

When the pattern of weakness and sensory loss affects more than one major nerve a lumbosacral plexus lesion should be suspected. The concurrent involvement of other plexal branches (i.e., gluteal nerves, posterior cutaneous nerve to the thigh, and/or pudendal nerve) helps confirm plexal injury. However, few testable nerve branches arise from the lumbosacral plexus, making lesion localization *within* the lumbosacral plexus difficult or impossible. The patient's history, risk factors, coexisting injuries, and mechanism of injury provide important information that should be used to help differentiate proximal branch injury versus true plexal damage. History of pelvic tumor, radiation, trauma, or a complicated delivery is especially pertinent. Aside from motor and sensory deficits, autonomic abnormalities, manifesting as erythematous, dry, warm skin, are often present with plexal injuries. Radiography, including plain X-rays, myelography, and computed tomographic myelography, is used to confirm fractures, pseudomeningoceles, hematomas, and foreign bodies, all of which aid lesion localization. Additionally, electromyography can help differentiate plexopathies, proximal mononeuropathies, and radiculopathies.

Lumbar plexus injuries manifest with hip flexion, hip adduction, and knee extension weakness. Sensory changes can occur in the lower abdomen (iliohypogastric nerve), groin (ilioinguinal nerve), genitalia/femoral triangle (genitofemoral nerve), lateral thigh (lateral femoral cutaneous nerve), anterior thigh (femoral nerve), medial thigh (femoral and obturator nerves), and medial lower leg down to the arch of the foot (saphenous nerve). Lumbar plexus injuries can be partial or complete. The most noticeable deficits with lumbar plexus damage are quadriceps weakness/wasting and anterior thigh sensory loss. For this reason, many patients with lumbar plexus damage are misdiagnosed as having only a femoral neuropathy. Therefore, it is important to remember that, for patients with complete or partial femoral palsies, one should check for adductor weakness (obturator nerve) and sensory loss on the anterolateral thigh (lateral femoral cutaneous nerve) to exclude a lumbar plexus injury.

Sacral plexus damage can cause sciatic nerve motor and sensory loss, sensory loss to the posterior midline thigh (posterior femoral cutaneous nerve), motor loss of the gluteal muscles (superior and inferior gluteal nerves), as well as sexual, bladder, and bowel dysfunction (pudendal nerve, autonomic nervous system). Analogous to a femoral nerve palsy from a lumbar plexus injury, sciatic nerve palsy is the predominant finding in sacral injury patients. Therefore, patients with suspected sciatic palsies, especially those with knee flexion weakness (hamstrings), should be fully evaluated for a sacral plexus injury. Evaluate sensation on the posterior thigh (posterior femoral cutaneous nerve), hip abduction and extension (superior and inferior gluteal nerves, respectively), and perianal sensation (pudendal nerve damage). Sacral plexus damage is difficult to differentiate from concurrent palsies of the sciatic, inferior gluteal, and posterior cutaneous nerves, all of which can be simultaneously injured distal to the plexus where they together exit the greater sciatic foramen below the pyriformis muscle. The superior gluteal and pudendal nerves exit the pelvis remote to these three nerves; therefore, hip abduction weakness and perineal sensory loss would be important findings that implicate a sacral plexus injury.

Focal damage to the lumbosacral trunk is particularly difficult to diagnose. L5 radiculopathy, lumbosacral trunk damage, sciatic nerve injury predominantly involving the common peroneal division, and common peroneal nerve palsy may all have a similar clinical presentation: foot drop. Lumbosacral trunk lesions may be differentiated from sciatic or common peroneal palsies because they often cause weakness in the posterior tibialis as well as other more proximal muscles, including the gluteals (hip extension and abduction). Differentiating an L5 radiculopathy from a lumbosacral trunk lesion is often not possible clinically. Imaging (to rule out nerve root compression) and electrodiagnostic testing (to document paraspinal muscle denervation) help confirm an L5 radiculopathy. A fracture/dislocation of the ipsilateral sacroiliac joint on computed tomographic scan or X-ray may point toward lumbosacral trunk damage in trauma patients with a foot drop.

Lower sacral plexus (S3–S5) damage causes perineal/perianal sensory loss, decreased anal sphincter tone, loss of an anal reflex, and loss of the bulbocavernosus reflex. Test the anal reflex (anal wink) by gently scratching the skin near the anus and observing the sphincter's reflexive contraction. Afferents for this reflex are carried by S5 and efferents by S3–S5. Test the bulbocavernosus reflex by briefly flicking the glans penis while your other hand palpates the bulbocavernosus muscle contraction behind the scrotum. Afferents for this reflex are carried by S3 and efferents by S3–S5.

Sympathetic fibers destined for the lower extremity originate from the upper lumbar spinal nerves and enter the sympathetic trunk to be subsequently distributed to the peripheral nerves in the lumbosacral plexus. Therefore, lumbosacral plexus and peripheral nerve (e.g., sciatic nerve) lesions can cause sympathetic abnormalities in the lower extremity (e.g., a warm, dry foot). In contrast, lower lumbar and sacral radiculopathies do not cause sympathetic abnormalities because the injury is proximal to where the sympathetic nerves join the plexus.

8.3.1 Spinal Nerve Dermatomes and Myotomes

Excluding a peripheral nerve problem in patients with presumed spinal radiculopathies is important, especially for surgical candidates without clear-cut back and radicular pain. This section provides a summary of the respective dermatomes and myotomes for the L1 to S1 spinal nerves. Overall, L2, L3, and L4 radiculopathies should be differentiated from femoral neuropathies, L5 radiculopathy from common peroneal nerve injury, and S1 radiculopathy from a tibial nerve lesion.

The *L1 spinal nerve* provides sensation to the hypogastric area, groin, and base of the penis/mons pubis. Muscle weakness does not occur. Of note, pain within the L1 dermatome is often nonneural in origin. Local processes, including hernias or lymphadenitis, are often the cause. Nonneural problems should not cause sensory loss, so if numbness is present, one should strongly consider local nerve injury, especially if the patient had previous groin surgery. Ilioinguinal, iliohypogastric, and genitofemoral neuropathies, as well as upper lumbar plexus lesions, are all in the differential diagnosis of a suspected L1 radiculopathy.

The *L2 spinal nerve* provides sensation to the anterior thigh and motor innervation to the iliopsoas muscle. Although both a femoral neuropathy and L2 radiculopathy may cause anterior thigh pain, numbness, or paresthesias, their motor deficits remain unique: femoral neuropathies cause quadriceps weakness; L2 radiculopathies cause iliopsoas weakness. Alternatively, if the motor exam is normal and spine imaging does not reveal a compressive lesion, anterolateral sensory loss on the thigh is likely meralgia paresthetica. For meralgia paresthetica the patellar reflex is normal.

The *L3 spinal nerve* provides sensation to the lower anterior thigh and knee region, along with motor innervation to the quadriceps and hip adductors. Therefore, the main differential of an L3 radiculopathy is also a femoral neuropathy. For patients with a femoral neuropathy, however, adductor strength would be normal, which is not the case for a severe L3 radiculopathy. Spine imaging and/or electrodiagnostic testing are required to differentiate an L3 radiculopathy from a lumbar plexus lesion.

The *L4 spinal nerve* carries sensation from the medial lower leg, in the saphenous nerve distribution. It provides substantial motor innervation to the quadriceps via the femoral nerve and the hip adductors via the obturator nerve. It also provides motor innervation to the anterior tibialis via the common peroneal nerve. To differentiate a femoral neuropathy from an L4 radiculopathy one should check for hip adductor and foot dorsiflexion weakness, which would be present only with a radiculopathy.

The *L5 spinal nerve* provides sensation to the anterolateral shin and dorsum of the foot. It also innervates all the muscles controlled by the common peroneal nerve. Therefore, a common peroneal neuropathy should be ruled out in all L5 radiculopathy patients. Fortunately, the L5 nerve root provides motor innervation to other muscles besides those innervated by the common peroneal nerve, including the posterior tibialis and glutei. Therefore, foot inversion (posterior tibialis) should be normal for patients with common peroneal lesions. Of note, patients with an L5 radiculopathy can have a depressed or absent ankle jerk; this is because large herniated disks at L4–L5 can also partially compress the S1 nerve root.

The *S1 spinal nerve* provides sensation to both the lateral aspect and sole of the foot via the sural and plantar nerves, respectively. Motor innervation includes the ankle flexors as well as all the foot intrinsics. This pattern of sensory and motor loss closely mimics that of the sciatic nerve's tibial division, and/or the tibial nerve itself. The S1 nerve root, however, also innervates the gluteal muscles via the superior and inferior gluteal nerves. Therefore, in addition to the presence of low back and radicular pain, gluteal weakness helps confirm an S1 radiculopathy. Furthermore, the posterior tibialis (L4, L5; foot inversion) does not receive S1 input, and therefore would be spared by an S1 radiculopathy, but not by a sciatic or tibial injury. A tibial neuropathy is further differentiated from both an S1 radiculopathy and a proximal sciatic lesion because it would spare both the gluteal muscles and the more proximally innervated hamstrings.

8.4 Processes Affecting the Lumbosacral Plexus

As with the brachial plexus, damage to the lumbosacral plexus can be categorized as structural or nonstructural. Structural etiologies include tumors, hemorrhage, surgery, obstetric/gynecologic procedures, trauma, and injections. Non-structural etiologies include lumbosacral amyotrophic neuralgia, radiation, vasculitis, diabetes, infection, and hereditary pressure palsies.

8.4.1 Trauma

Traumatic lumbosacral plexopathy is often partial and mostly caused by high-speed deceleration (i.e., motor vehicle) accidents where the pelvis or hip is fractured/dislocated. In fact, about one quarter of all pelvic fractures are associated with nerve damage, plexal or otherwise. Most traumatic lumbosacral plexus injuries are postganglionic, secondary to stretch or traction. However, sacroiliac joint fractures or dislocations may actually cause spinal nerve avulsion. These avulsions can occur in or out of the spinal canal. As in the cervical region, myelography and magnetic resonance imaging assist with the diagnosis of nerve avulsion by documenting pseudomeningoceles. Considering the proximity of the lumbosacral trunk to the sacroiliac joint, it may be selectively damaged with fracture/dislocations in this area. Because the lumbosacral trunk carries nerves destined for the common peroneal division of the sciatic nerve, these patients present with a foot drop.

For classification, traumatic and iatrogenic injury of the lumbosacral plexus may be divided into four diagnostic zones, with most patients having more then one zone either completely or partially involved. Zone 1 involves the anterior divisions of the lumbar plexus (the obturator nerve; medial thigh). Zone 2 involves the posterior divisions of the lumbar plexus (the femoral and lateral femoral cutaneous nerves; anterior, medial, and lateral thigh/leg). Zone 3 refers to the anterior divisions of the sacral plexus (the tibial division of the sciatic nerve). Zone 4 involves the posterior divisions of the sacral plexus (the common peroneal division of the sciatic nerve as well as the superior and inferior gluteal nerves). The clinical utility of this zone-based categorization of lumbosacral injuries is limited because most injuries do not follow these convenient boundaries. Preliminary data reveal that trauma most frequently involves either the sacral plexus alone or the complete lumbosacral plexus. Isolated, traumatic lumbar plexus injuries are rare.

8.4.2 Retroperitoneal Hemorrhage

Coagulopathic patients may have spontaneous retroperitoneal hemorrhages. Patients with normal clotting may also have retroperitoneal bleeds following trauma, retroperitoneal surgery, or groin catheterization. Hemorrhage may be confined to the psoas muscle, iliacus muscle, or abdominal wall; larger hemorrhages may involve all three. A psoas muscle hemorrhage would selectively compress the lumbar plexus. These patients have acute, often severe, back pain radiating to their groin and anterior thigh. Weakness occurs in the quadriceps, iliopsoas, and, occasionally, the hip adductors. Severe pain may limit the accuracy of the neurological assessment. There may be sensory loss in a lumbar plexus distribution, mostly the groin and anterior thigh. Hip movement is painful, and patients are often only comfortable when the hip is flexed.

Extensive hemorrhages affecting the lumbar plexus can also track caudally to compress the lumbosacral trunk and sacral plexus. Alternatively, focal hemorrhages in the iliacus muscle (i.e., iliacus compartment), which typically can occur following groin catheterization, may selectively compress the femoral nerve.

8.4.3 Lumbosacral Plexitis (Amyotrophic Neuralgia)

This clinical ailment of uncertain etiology can affect the lumbosacral plexus like it does the brachial plexus. Patients present with acute or subacute onset of proximal lower-extremity pain, often radiating down the anteromedial or posterior thigh, sometimes into the lower leg. The pain is quite severe and limits motor assessment. Days to weeks later (on average one week), weakness appears in the distribution of the pain. Paresthesias may also occur. Plexal involvement is usually partial, affecting either multiple plexal branches or just one (e.g., the femoral nerve). Over time, the pain and weakness slowly resolve, with some patients having near complete resolution after several months.

8.4.4 Proximal Diabetic Neuropathy

Weakness is the predominant manifestation of proximal diabetic neuropathy (diabetic amyotrophy). It usually causes hip flexion, hip adduction, hip abduction, and knee extension weakness (femoral, obturator, and gluteal nerves). Atrophy of the proximal thigh and hip girdle may occur. Although pain can be severe, concentrated in the back, groin, or anteromedial thigh, many patients have only mild or no pain. As with idiopathic lumbosacral plexitis, weakness and pain from proximal diabetic neuropathy usually resolve in several months to a year. Residual stiffness and weakness can persist, however. Acute diabetic neuropathies affecting only the femoral nerve are quite rare; most patients actually have other, perhaps subtle, involvement of the lumbar plexus. The etiology of proximal diabetic neuropathy may be epineurial microvasculitis.

Two distinct types of proximal diabetic neuropathy can occur. The first type is descriptively called *proximal asymmetric neuropathy*. Patients with this type have abrupt onset of unilateral weakness as well as severe inguinal and thigh pain. Patients report trouble ambulating because of knee buckling. Diabetic patients with this type usually do not have peripheral (stocking-glove) neuropathy and are not insulin dependent. A history of recent weight loss, curiously, is often present.

The second type is called *proximal symmetrical neuropathy*. It often occurs in insulin-dependent diabetics with a history of peripheral (stocking-glove) neuropathy. The onset of weakness is slow, manifesting over days to weeks. The weakness is bilateral and somewhat asymmetrical (despite the name). Pain can occur but is slow in onset.

8.4.5 Neoplastic and Radiation Damage

Pelvic tumors may cause plexopathy, with severe pain, not weakness, as the primary complaint. The initial presentation is usually an insidious onset of back or pelvic pain that radiates to the thigh or leg. Weakness and/or numbness can occur, but these deficits are usually minimal. If the tumor involves the most caudal fibers of the sacral plexus bilaterally, incontinence can also occur. Primary tumors affecting the lumbosacral plexus include colorectal, uterine, prostate, and ovarian tumors. Secondary, or metastatic, tumors involving the lumbosacral plexus include breast, sarcoma, lymphoma, testicular, and thyroid tumors. Malignant invasion of the lumbosacral plexus has four patterns: lumbosacral involvement only, sacral plexus involvement only, complete ipsilateral lumbosacral plexus involvement, and bilateral lower sacral involvement.

Pelvic, or lower paraspinal, radiation therapy may also cause lumbosacral plexopathy. Radiation doses > 5,000 rad are usually required, with symptoms appearing slowly, on average 5 years later (range, 1–30 years). Radiation plex-opathy is usually painless, or with minimal pain, which is a key finding that helps differentiate radiation plexopathy from infiltrative, recurrent tumor, which is usually painful. Radiation plexopathy presents with an insidious onset of weakness. The rate of progression and completeness of the deficit are variable. The majority of cases are bilateral. Numbness and paresthesias may occur. Weakness often stabilizes once it is profound. Improvement is unlikely. Myokymic discharges on needle electromyography occur in radiation plexopathy, being a useful way to confirm the diagnosis.

Index

Note: Pages numbers followed by f indicate figures; t tables.